Books by Cynthia Olsen

Looking Up: Seven Steps for a Healthy & Youthful Midlife and Beyond

Australian Tea Tree Oil Guide (1st ed.)

Australian Tea Tree Oil Guide (2nd ed.), also available in Spanish

Australian Tea Tree Oil Handbook: 101 Ways to Use Australian Tea Tree Oil (1st Ed.)

Australian Tea Tree Oil Handbook: 101 Plus Ways to Use Australian Tea Tree Oil (2nd ed.)

Essiac: A Native Herbal Cancer Remedy (2nd ed.)

Birth of the Blue: Australian Blue Cypress Oil

Awards and Testimonials

IPPY GOLD BOOK AWARD

LIVING NOW SILVER BOOK AWARD

USA BOOK AWARD FINALIST

SW BOOK FINALIST

I have thought for much of my life that health is far more important than life itself. There are many approaches to living the healthy life, but the key is DOING the essentials. Those seven essentials are clearly described in *Looking Up*. Now your only need is to DO THEM!

—C Norman Shealy,
MD, PhD

Looking Up is a wonderful title for a GREAT way to live your life: simple solutions to connect to yourself and live healthily.

—Mariel Hemingway,
Actor, Author, Activist

Looking Up is filled with information that we should all know about. Cynthia has shared her wisdom on health, vitality, and living well in this comprehensive and easy to understand book. This book is must-read. If you feel as though you already lead a healthy lifestyle, you'll learn something new, and if you are just beginning down a path toward wellness, pick up this book. You'll find it to be a wonderful guide!

—Susan Engle,
MSOM, LAC

Looking Up is a resource guide for the habits of those in search of a rich life. It helped me take all of the learning of many great books and synthesize it into one book. The information in the book shares the "secrets" to be the most vibrant and joyful person you can be. As a former public educator and a present-day reflexologist, I believe what Cynthia says, "share life's experiences in health and mindfulness which are guideposts for everyday living."

—Theresa Carullo,
Reflexologist

It is possible for you to grow younger—and Cynthia Olsen provides a remarkable amount of information for you to start the process right now.

—Ellen Wood,
Grow Young Guide and
author of *Think and Grow Young*

What a great book. I can't imagine all the research and time that went into writing it. You certainly have covered all bases with easy to understand and useful information for mental as well as physical health. Many of your recommendations on diet and exercise are what I teach to my patients. Good luck with your book. I know it will benefit many readers.

—Donald Cuccia,
MD, Internal Medicine

Embracing YOUR Age

CYNTHIA OLSEN

Embracing Your Age
Feeling Vibrant at Every Stage of Your Life

Disclaimer: The information provided in this book is strictly for informational purposes and is not intended as a substitute for advice from your physician or mental health provider. You should not use this information for diagnosis or treatment of any physical or mental health problem.

In this world of digital information and rapidly-changing technology, some citations do not provide exact page numbers or credit the original source. We regret any errors, which are a result of the ease with which we consume information.

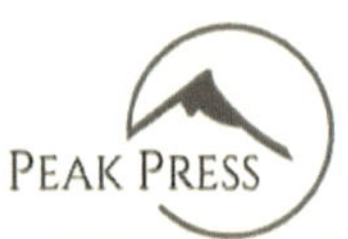

An Imprint for GracePoint Publishing (www.GracePointPublishing.com)

GracePoint Matrix, LLC
624 S. Cascade Ave, Suite 201
Colorado Springs, CO 80903
www.GracePointMatrix.com
Email: Admin@GracePointMatrix.com
SAN # 991-6032

Library of Congress Control Number: 2023939104

ISBN: (Paperback) 978-0-9893336-1-0
eISBN: 978-0-9893336-2-7

Books may be purchased for educational, business, or sales promotional use.
For bulk order requests and price schedule contact:
Orders@GracePointPublishing.com

Dedication

I dedicate this book to my grandparents and parents, who were my outstanding teachers and who instilled in me core values which have sustained me throughout my lifetime.

To my sister Patricia and my beautiful daughter Tamara who left us too soon.

To the next generation, my children, grandchildren, and great-grandchildren, my love for you is everlasting. My wish for you—long and healthy lives.

To my great-nephew Joe who has taught our family the true meaning of love. His attitude of gratitude has given him the ability to conquer his limitations.

To Sharon and Bob—God bless you.

I also dedicate this book to the fellowship of my far-reaching extended family that has touched my life with love, support, and encouragement.

To all of you I am eternally grateful.

Table of Contents

Prefazione

La Carta presentata trent'anni fa alla prima Conferenza Internazionale sulla Promozione della Salute riunitasi a Ottawa, definisce la promozione della salute "il processo che mette in grado le persone di aumentare il controllo sulla propria salute e di migliorarla" (WHO, 1986). La salute è intesa non come obiettivo dell'esistenza, ma come una vera e propria risorsa, che consente agli individui di realizzare i propri progetti di vita. Promuovere la salute significa aiutare le persone a sviluppare quelle abilità che consentono loro di affrontare le sfide della vita quotidiana, e prendere responsabilmente decisioni. Promuovere la salute significa anche rendere i contesti ambientali di vita e di lavoro favorevoli alle scelte salutari. Gli individui e i gruppi possono diventare soggetti attivi nel perseguire uno stato di buona salute quando sono in grado di riconoscere e soddisfare i propri bisogni, di modificare l'ambiente o di adattarvisi sviluppando qualità resilienti. Da questo punto di vista la promozione della salute è responsabilità di tutti i settori (sanità, istruzione, cultura, agricoltura, economia, ecc.) che influiscono sui determinanti della salute. Stili di vita, condizioni socio economiche e ambiente hanno il maggior peso nel determinare lo stato di salute.

Le patologie croniche come le malattie cardiache e l'ipertensione, alcuni tipi di cancro, il diabete di tipo 2, le malattie respiratorie croniche rappresentano oggi un allarme planetario con circa 38 milioni di morti ogni anno. Riguardo agli stili di vita le linee guida internazionali (WHO, 2004), danno, tra l'altro, le seguenti indicazioni :

Praticare un' attività fisica regolare, d'intensità moderata, per almeno

30 minuti al giorno, 5 giorni a settimana

Limitare l'aggiunta di sale ai cibi (nella nostra comune alimentazione, il sodio contenuto in natura negli alimenti, è già sufficiente a coprire il fabbisogno dell'organismo di questo elemento)

Incrementare il consumo di frutta e verdura (almeno 5 porzioni al giorno), legumi, cereali integrali e frutta secca

Astenersi dal fumo

L'attività fisica inoltre è utile a prevenire le demenze che rappresentano oggi un serio problema in età avanzata. Il nostro corpo infatti è nato e "costruito" per il movimento e stare otto ore seduti a una scrivania richiama a gran voce di inserire nella giornata un sano esercizio fisico.

Nelle pagine di questo libro, Cynthia va oltre i suggerimenti sugli stili di vita consapevoli perché fornisce spunti su come si può *generare* benessere, non si limita infatti a proporre una vita dinamica, socialmente appagante, nutrizionalmente adeguata, ma prospetta in che modo poter rafforzare le proprie abilità personali (cognitive, emotive, relazionali) e le reti sociali per affrontare le sfide della vita quotidiana e "produrre" il benessere proprio e nella comunità. Il punto di vista sulla salute è quello di risorsa per coltivare le proprie passioni e vivere consapevolmente il momento presente per sentirsi rafforzato dal proprio passato, anche doloroso, (questa è resilienza!), e motivato a progettare e realizzare i propri progetti di vita. Qui l'età non conta! "Forget your age :Live now!" L'autore inoltre esorta a essere soggetti attivi, protagonisti della propria salute, con attenzione rispettosa dell'ambiente e con un modo di vivere sobrio che dà giusta dignità a chi è meno fortunato nell'accedere a quanto noi ci possiamo permettere (cibo, cure, abitazioni confortevoli, serenità economica, istruzione ecc.).

A mio avviso il libro può essere piacevolmente letto in due modi. Il primo è quello di scoprire i sette step in modo progressivo per individuare e immagazzinare tutte le piccole luci che riteniamo utili a illuminare il corso della nostra vita. E' preso in considerazione come prendersi cura della mente, del corpo, dell'alimentazione (anche usando integratori dopo appropriata informazione medica), della pelle, delle nostre finanze e come vivere consapevolmente il momento presente.

Il secondo è quello di andare per ordine d'interesse, partendo dallo step che adesso ci attrae di più per balzare poi, con curiosità, alla scoperta degli altri come in un'avventura alla ricerca dei piccoli tesori da mettere nella bisaccia perché possano servirci a migliorare il nostro ben-essere.

C'è ancora un punto di forza che tengo a sottolineare. I temi dei capitoli, scritti con un linguaggio divulgativo, di lettura scorrevole, sono resi concreti dal racconto di esperienze di vita personali e dall'utilizzo di riferimenti scientifici. I suggerimenti per ogni step inseriti negli elenchi schematici consentono un'agevole e chiara individuazione.

Non posso nascondere che gli episodi di vita con i nonni italiani, la tavola imbandita con i prodotti della dieta mediterranea, mi hanno commosso nella stessa misura con la quale trovandosi in un Paese straniero ci illuminiamo quando incontriamo un nostro connazionale. La dieta mediterranea che contribuisce a prevenire le malattie croniche legate all'alimentazione per il momento sta ancora resistendo nel nostro Paese anche se assistiamo a cambiamenti alimentari dovuti alla globalizzazione.

Infine, aver inserito da parte dell'autore la propria storia in questo libro ne rende ancora più prezioso il contenuto, perché crea con il lettore una sintonia legata al cuore.

Queste pagine non sono solo da leggere, ma soprattutto da vivere. Pienamente. Nel momento presente. Grazie Cynthia.

Margherita Brunetti, MD, è specializzata in Igiene e Medicina Preventiva orientamento Sanità Pubblica presso l'Università di Pisa (Italia). Nella stessa Università ha conseguito il Master di primo livello in Comunicazione Bio-Sanitaria. Dal 1988 lavora nell'ambito della Sanità Pubblica e si è occupata prevalentemente di sicurezza alimentare, nutrizione e promozione di sani stili di vita. Da cinque anni è responsabile dell'educazione e promozione della salute nel territorio pisano. E' Presidente della Delegazione Toscana della Società Italiana di Promozione della Salute. E' Trainer in Tecniche di Transformative Mindfulness per il controllo del dolore e della sofferenza. Attualmente si sta perfezionando per conseguire il Master Universitario di Istruttore facilitatore di protocolli basati sulla Mindfulness e Pratiche Contemplative.

Sitografia

http://www.who.int/healthpromotion/conferences/previous/ottawa/en/

Foreword

The Paper presented thirty years ago at the First International Conference on Health Promotion in Ottawa defines *Health Promotion* as "the process of enabling people to increase control over, and to improve, their health" (WHO, 1986). Health is not intended as the goal of existence, but as a resource that allows individuals to achieve their long-term life plans. Promoting health means to help people develop skills that better help them face the challenges of everyday life and make responsible choices. It also means to build work and home environments that are favorable to healthy choices. When individuals and groups have the chance to figure out and satisfy their own needs, or when they can modify their own environments or adapt to them by developing resiliency, they become active subjects in the pursuit of being well. From this point of view, health promotion is a responsibility of all sectors (health, instruction, culture, agriculture, economy, etc.) that influence health determinants. Lifestyles, socioeconomic conditions, and environment are the most significant factors in determining health status.

Today chronic pathologies, such as heart disease, hypertension, some varieties of cancer, type 2 diabetes, and chronic breathing disorders represent a planetary concern, with about thirty-eight million deaths every year. Regarding lifestyles, the international guidelines (WHO, 2004) provide the following indications:

- Practice consistent physical activity, at moderate intensity, at least thirty minutes a day, five days a week
- Limit the addition of salt to foods (the amount of sodium naturally present in our nourishment is already enough to satisfy our body's need for it)
- Increase consumption of fruit and vegetables (at least five servings a day), legumes, integral cereals, and dried fruit

- No smoking

Physical activity is also useful to prevent dementia, which nowadays represents a serious issue in seniors. This is because our bodies have been "built" to move, so sitting at a desk for eight hours begs for some healthy physical exercise to be added to our day.

In the pages of this book, the author goes beyond giving advice on conscious lifestyles, because she provides ideas on how to generate well-being. She doesn't limit herself to promoting a dynamic, socially fulfilling, and nutritionally adequate life, and instead outlines how to strengthen one's own personal skills (cognitive, emotional, relational) and all social interactions to face the challenges of everyday life, and how to craft well-being for oneself and in the community. She sees health as a resource to cultivate one's own interests and to live knowingly in the present moment in order to feel empowered by the past, even when painful (this is resiliency!) and motivated to plan and realize long-term life goals. Age doesn't matter! "Forget your age: Live now!" The author also urges us to be active subjects, protagonists of our own health, with respectful concern for the environment and by leading a balanced and moderate way of living that is fair to those who are less privileged and can't afford all the things we can (food, care, living conditions, financial stability, instruction, etc.).

I believe that this book can be enjoyed and read in two ways. The first way is to discover the seven steps progressively, to understand and save them for later as tiny lights that we will need to illuminate the journey of our lives. This includes taking good care of our minds and bodies, our nutrition (even by using supplements, after receiving the appropriate medical information), our skin, and our finances, and living in awareness in the present moment.

The second way is to follow your own level of interest, starting from the step that sounds more appealing, and jump later, with curiosity, to discover all the others, like in an adventure—hunting little treasures that we can keep in our purses as tools to improve our well-being.

There is one more strong point that I want to underline. The topics of the chapters, written with straightforward and smooth laypeople's language, are solidified by the tales of personal experiences and the commitment to scientific references. The advice for each step, listed schematically, is clear and easy to locate.

I can't deny that the stories about the Italian grandparents, the laid table with the products of the Mediterranean diet, moved me in the same way we light up when we are in a foreign land, and we meet a compatriot. The Mediterranean diet, which contributes to prevent nutrition-based chronic diseases, is still holding up in our country even though we are seeing dietary changes due to globalization.

Finally, by making her own personal story part of this book the author made its content even more precious, as that creates a harmony with the reader that is based on the heart.

These pages shouldn't just be read, they should be lived. In full. In the present moment.

Thank you, Cynthia.

Margerita Brunetti

Margerita Brunetti, MD, specializes in hygiene and preventive medicine in the context of public health at the University of Pisa (Italy). In the same university she achieved a first level master's degree in bio-sanitary communication. Since 1988 she has been working in public health and focuses her attention on food safety, nutrition, and promotion of healthy lifestyles. In the last five years she has been responsible for health promotion and education in the area of Pisa. She is president of the Tuscan Delegation of the Italian Health Promotion Society. She is also a trainer in transformative mindfulness techniques for the control of pain and suffering, and at the present moment she is about to achieve a master's degree to become an instructor and facilitator for protocols based on mindfulness and contemplative practices.

Webography

http://www.who.int/healthpromotion/conferences/previous/ottawa/en/

Introduction

Wake up! If you knew for certain that you had a terminal illness... if you had little time left to live—you would waste precious little of it! Well, I'm telling you... you do have a terminal illness: It's called birth. You don't have more than a few years left. No one does! So be happy now, without reason—or you never will be at all.

—*Dan Millman*
The Way of the Peaceful Warrior

When I was growing up my grandmother Jennie used to tell me, "When you have your health, you have everything." She should know, having lost a leg to diabetes mellitus type 2 in her sixties and then learning to walk again in spite of all the adversities. She would repeat the phrase quite often; perhaps it became the mantra that gave her courage and strength to get up each morning, put on her prosthesis, and go about her daily life. She survived into her upper seventies, passing away in her sleep. Her resilience and attitude, coupled with faith in herself and God, gave her a longer life than the doctors predicted. She outlived her husband and one of her daughters, my mother.

I had a healthy start in my own life. I grew up in an Italian American family with both maternal and paternal grandparents who had been born in Italy, so I followed a Mediterranean diet long before it became *en vogue*. My mother prepared fresh, wholesome food, and what a difference fresh food makes.

We always had a variety of yogurt, vegetables, dairy, and meat on hand.

Milk was delivered in glass bottles with thick cream floating on the top. There were no genetically modified foods back then.

Sugar, however, was everywhere. During the holidays, we enjoyed luscious (and rich) Italian baked goods. Life was delicious. My grandmother Jennie was addicted to sugar. She stashed sweets in a hideout in the pantry. When her diabetes got worse, I believe she regretted not having more willpower to overcome her sugar addiction.

My parents were not physically active people, and as a result their health was compromised as they grew older, something I witnessed firsthand. My mother developed rheumatoid arthritis (RA) and my dad, kidney disease. My mother suffered ongoing aches in her thirties. Her hands and feet were so badly crippled she couldn't open a jar or fit her swollen feet into shoes. She spent many years depressed and in pain. My father looked after her, and the daily stress took a terrible toll on his well-being too.

As children, my siblings and I were careful to monitor our behavior based on whether my mother's bedroom door was closed during the day, which indicated she was resting. My dad was always trying to compensate for my mother's forced inactivity by taking us on sojourns into the city or Sunday drives in the car. She had no desire to exercise or go to therapy—especially after falling and breaking her hip at age forty-five. Her medical doctor and the National Institutes of Health wanted to run more extensive research on her because of her severe RA; however, she refused just as she seemed to refuse taking more positive steps to improve her health. Some winter days my father would find her hanging clothes outside, which would only make her joints swell and send her to bed. My mother tried to control everything around her. I read once that people who suffer with RA possess a rigid manner in their life. I often wondered if there was a correlation between that and my mother's RA. As far as we can determine, there hasn't been any other family member diagnosed with RA. After years of ill health, my mother developed lupus and died of a stroke at fifty-three. I was twenty-six at the time. My dad passed away six weeks later, at sixty-three; his death is still unexplained. I think he died of a broken heart.

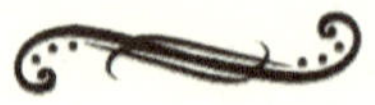

I have always thrived on being active—swimming at three, tennis, baseball, basketball, roller skating, hiking, canoeing, biking, horseback riding—you name it. So as I get older, it's been like second nature to incorporate more activity into my days. However, I was not yet sitting still long enough to rest; that was a challenge for me. In my twenty's and halfway into my thirty's, I was raising my five very active children, and I didn't yet know and understand the spiritual side of life. I had occasional flashes of insight and the feeling that there was a good deal more for me to learn about my spiritual side, but there was little time to contemplate these feelings while meeting the demands of my family.

Into my thirties I began to read books by Carlos Castaneda, a Peruvian author who wrote about his teacher, a Yaqui shaman named Don Juan Matus, whom he met in 1960. The teacher taught him the ways of a Yaqui warrior. I expanded my yearnings for more in-depth spiritual knowledge through *The Prophet*, by Kahlil Gibran, and explored psychic writings by Jane Roberts—*Seth Speaks,* among others. Jane was considered one of the leading psychics in the twentieth century. She would often go into a trance and write about her communications. She lived within an hour of us in upper New York State when I was twenty-five. My friend was her neighbor and told me we could come to her place and participate in a spiritual meeting, but I was naive at the time, and had little interest in meeting her. Perhaps it wasn't the time for me to explore this area even though the Ouija board became constant entertainment for us.

I quit smoking cigarettes when I was twenty-eight, before the Surgeon General's report on the hazards of tobacco. My sixth sense told me that inhaling tobacco would eventually compromise my health in some way. I also cut back on alcohol at around the same time, as the two habits seemed to go hand in hand.

My parents had the foresight to ship my siblings and me off to camp during the summer months. In the Adirondack Mountains, where I spent most of my early years, the air and lakes seemed especially clean during the 1950s. I swam in our lake along with the fish, turtles, and water plants. We didn't talk about global warming back then, nor did we see any evidence of pollution, although acid rain eventually destroyed most of the flora and fish. The days were bright and clear, and the evening sky was filled with a magnificent showing of the Northern Lights.

We were raised in the Catholic Church, but as I grew up, I pulled away, seeking alternative spiritual avenues. I began to practice yoga when I was in my midthirties and made friends who talked about metaphysics and what it meant to be psychic. I began to find ways to balance my days, to become more peaceful and to better handle stress. I lived in the Colorado mountains and would seek out solitude through hikes into the wilderness areas. In the winter, I cross-country skied on trails away from the tourists. I cooked healthy foods, not unlike the Mediterranean diet I grew up with. I read every label on the supermarket shelves. I started to experiment with cooking tofu and digging my hands into a garden of vegetables. I frequented farmers' markets for fresh fruits and produce. I made healthy school lunches of organic peanut butter spread on luscious whole grain bread. My world back then seemed like a laboratory, with me as the mad chemist; everyone within my reach became my guinea pig.

I look back on that period of my life as my education in health, even though I wasn't totally conscious of it. I purchased healthy recipe cookbooks; *Laura in the Kitchen* became my kitchen bible. The children sometimes questioned what they were eating, but I persevered. My youngest stepson wasn't used to eating healthy food and at dinner would run to the bathroom to throw up. I was extremely grateful that he didn't continue this ritual. Sometimes for dessert I would bake a yummy cheesecake made with tofu and fresh fruit. At first, they would express amazement that I made such a dessert until they were told its ingredients. They seemed to be ok with the healthier version. Nutrition has been an ongoing journey in my life. Genetically modified foods (GMO), herbicides, and pesticides, processed foods, hormone injected beef, chickens raised under unsanitary conditions, to name just a few, have invaded our planet since I grew into adulthood, so I became watchful in the types of food to prepare.

My many gardens were experimental. In the mountains I would haul my neighbor's animal manure down the road to prepare my garden for planting. My daughter's horse escaped one day and I had to chase him away before he ate all of the lettuce. During my twenty's we lived in Southern Florida on an acre of land. I rented a rototiller to prepare the garden. I was a novice so decided to plant radishes to begin with. In spring, we had a variety of red, white, and hot radishes growing among a few bunches of lettuce. The avocado, banana, and mango trees on our property provided us with fresh fruit.

What I've learned from all the people and experiences I've had is that my life has always presented opportunities for me to have steppingstones to grow, and those simple changes, especially when presented in times of adversity, made a big difference. We are all born with a finite set of genes, but they are only one factor in our health among many—and the only one that we can't control in some way. I have walked the major avenues to longevity and vitality—nutrition, exercise, positive relationships, quality health care, geographic location, financial well-being, the mind-body connection, and avoiding alcohol, tobacco, and drugs. I want to pass along what I've learned so others can also be vibrant at any age.

Learning about life is always present for me. I write about Bruce Lipton and epigenetics in the mind section of this book. Bruce was a medical professor at the University of Wisconsin years back. He has researched and written books on the subject of epigenetics and how it plays a major role in her well-being; the genes playing a smaller part than we have been told. Our environment, emotional well-being, beliefs and culture all play a part in living a full and empowered life.

Research has shown that the attitudes of our mind can create disease or wellness. I write about my mother and her RA and how she resigned herself to living as an invalid in her midforties until her death at fifty-three years of age. My mother needed to control and have perfection in her world. As children, we were not permitted to rearrange or live in certain areas of our home. My father designed and built a finished recreational area in our basement where we could play. Perfection has been shown to be the root of many illnesses. My heritage doesn't show anyone who had RA. Throughout childhood, we are bombarded with subconscious patterning, be it betrayal, shame, or abandonment issues. As we age, we carry negative thought forms unless we have learned to recognize and heal our subconscious patterns. How often do you hear negative conversations around you? I'm too old to learn new things, or I have this illness which I can do nothing about, or I'm not fit to walk or travel. Healthy centurions (over 100) are future oriented, rebels, and not co-dependent. They hang around in clusters of like-minded people that support their agelessness thinking.

Dr. Masaru Emoto's book *The Hidden Messages in Water,* says, "we must pay respect to water, feel love and gratitude, and receive vibrations with a positive attitude. Then, water changes, you change, and I change, because both you and I are water" (Emoto, 2001). Dr. Emoto collected water samples from around the world and, after exposing the samples to visual words and music, he froze the water samples. The result showed that positive energy created beautiful crystal shapes, while the negative showed ugly ones.

It's important to recognize the body, mind, and spirit connection. Nutritious food, physical exercise, visualization, stress reduction, meditation along with a balanced, sharp mind, and peaceful and grateful nature, gets one in touch with the vital energy force of one's being. Please read my story with a discerning eye. Educate yourself so that you can discover the direction which most closely "resonates" with you for your particular life. In other words, follow your heart—your own intuition. These are the ways to luminescent living and being the most vibrant and joyful person you can be at any age. My desires and my prayers are to communicate this knowledge to you in a way that sparks your entire being and feeds your soul.

Step 1

Mind, Attitude, and Health—The Benefits

Mind is the master power that moulds and makes,
And man is mind, and evermore he takes
The tool of thought, and shaping what he wills,
Brings forth a thousand joys, a thousand ills.

—James Allen

While researching information for this book, I was reminded that a healthy life includes how our mind perceives things and how we react to the world around us. It's about eating healthy foods and surrounding ourselves with good friends and a nurturing family. Of course, we don't have control over other people's actions—unless their actions are causing us physical or mental harm. So, controlling the world around us means controlling our inner world. So, how can we do this?

One important discovery I've made along the line is is the importance of getting to know my true self. What does this mean? I am not easily influenced by what I hear from others or read in the newspaper or watch on television. When I was injured, I heard some people say "so debilitating" and "it's going to take you a long time to recover," but I refused to be influenced by someone else's opinion of me and my current situation. It is vital for me to seek my own truths in order for me to become my true self.

If we are faced with an illness or an accident, how do we choose to address it? Suppose we have been told we have cancer and the only way to fight it is through chemotherapy, radiation, and drugs. That is precisely what my sister was told by her doctor. She tried to cure herself in Africa by taking a native brew. She went to Cuban women in Florida who prepared herbs for her. When none of this helped, she took the traditional route as the doctors prescribed. She informed me that if she didn't do this she would die. During treatment, she became violently sick and weak. The cancer spread, and she died several months later. My sister never believed she would get well. She became desperate and refused to stop working until the day her strength gave out. Fear took over her life.

In my own life and since my accident, I have realized that my mind may have played an even larger part than I realized in my overall health and healing. I had a compound fracture and was in another country being treated. My doctor in Colorado had concerns that I could develop a bone disease from the fall, especially because it was exposed, if the immediate medical treatment wasn't performed properly in Nassau. I refused to imagine that would be happening to me. So, while flying home, which was a very long trip, I prayed and sent positive energy to my injury which gave me calmness and peace. My tolerance for pain increased, and I was more capable of handling my situation with less stress and a clearer mind.

Creating Positive Attitudes Along with Healthy Habits Can Make Us Truly Happier People

"Happiness is 50 percent genetic, and the rest is up to us," says David Lykken, a University of Minnesota researcher. (This is also said by others.) To many, happiness doesn't come from being rich and prosperous or owning things. Take in life's small pleasures, make an effort to stay healthy, and focus your energy inward instead of outward. Create and sustain meaningful relationships with family and friends. Consider engaging in a worthwhile philanthropic endeavor or connecting with your church.

Author Gregg Easterbrook writes, "Research shows that people who are grateful, optimistic, and forgiving have better experiences with their lives; more happiness, fewer strokes, and higher incomes. If you are looking for something to complain about, you are absolutely certain to find it. It requires some effort to achieve a happy outlook on life and most people don't make it. Most people take the path of least resistance. Far too many people today don't make the steps to make their life more fulfilling" (2006).

Heart disease is the number one killer in the United States, accounting for more than 40 percent of all deaths annually. A study done by the National Institute on Aging involved 229 Chicago-area men and women, ages fifty to sixty-eight. It showed that people who say they are lonely have higher blood pressure, which contributes to heart disease. Their systolic blood pressure was ten to thirty points higher than average. Harvard and Duke Universities found a similar result in people who isolated themselves. Based on these findings, it appears that not only do we need other people for survival, we need them for longevity and well-being. I live alone and yet I am not lonely. I surround myself with a supportive and loving network of family and friends. I participate in activities that include other like-minded individuals.

Doctors have long acknowledged the influence our thought patterns have on the body, but usually only among themselves. First-year medical texts sometimes admit that as much as 50 percent of disease is psychosomatic; in other words, "of the mind." Many physicians may fear admitting that much disease is rooted in the mind would put them out of business, leaving only psychiatrists to practice medicine.

Recently, however, we are hearing a few forthright MDs actually speaking publicly about the effect of one's thoughts upon the physical body. Take, for instance, the placebo effect. According to a French psychiatrist, Patrick Lemoine, almost 40 percent of pills prescribed by doctors are impure, meaning that they only contain a small amount of medicine in a sugar pill which doesn't medically assist the patient in getting better. Yet the doctor prescribes the pill, and the patient's mind believes there will be an improvement. There are many cases of placebo effects on patients with heart disease as well as Parkinson's. Another more extreme case of mind over matter is the remarkable story of a Spanish doctor, Angel Escudero, who has performed over 900 surgeries without anesthesia. Dr. Escudero performed surgery on a woman who had a severe leg deformity. By making sure her mouth was lubricated with her own saliva and telling herself she was anesthetized, her brain relaxed, and the pain receptors were turned off.

In China, medical doctors have long applied acupuncture, a two-thousand-year-old method of inserting needles in various parts of the body. In 1958 acupuncture was used to block pain receptors during surgery to remove tonsils.

Mao Tse Tung, the Chinese leader, mandated that all medical procedures were to be done using acupuncture rather than anesthesia. Acupuncture can divert feelings of pain; however, other sensations may be felt. Today, Chinese doctors use acupuncture primarily on head and neck surgeries.

The eloquent and increasingly popular Dr. Deepak Chopra tells how an individual thought can instantly impact the body via the creation of a neurotransmitter or hormone. Norman Cousins, author of *Anatomy of an Illness*, was diagnosed in 1964 with Ankylosing Spondylitis (crippling collagen disease). His doctor gave him a one in 500 chance of recovery. After a series of standard hospital procedures, Cousins checked himself out of the hospital and moved into a hotel. He believed that positive attitudes would result in positive results. Surrounding himself with funny movies and alternative healing methods such as intravenous vitamin C therapy, he made a full recovery. After reading Dr. Cousin's story, I thought back to my mother. How much did emotions play a part in her RA, immune system, and health? During the 1960s, psychiatrist George Solomon was an early pioneer in psychoneuroimmunology (PNI), the study of mind/body connection. He observed the connection between depression and people with RA, noting that their depression seemed to make their condition worse.

Dr. David Felton, neurobiologist of the University of Rochester School of Medicine and expert in the field of PNI, has made a remarkable discovery linking the immune system and central nervous system together—all of which is controlled by the brain. A network of nerves from our brain sends signals to the cells of the immune system, producing the body/mind connection. Attitudes, feelings, and emotions can have a direct bearing on the immune system.

An Arizona physician, Robert Koppen, MD, stated that results in the physical world happened because thought and feeling together were combined with creative energy. He went on to express that this concept did not have to be believed to be true. Further, he believed the mind-body connection a double-edged sword in that those who are happy and at peace are able to magnify and ignite beauty and the Divine intelligence; but the flip is also true: Feeling, expressing, and complaining about the negatives of life may destroy mental, emotional, and physical health by perpetuating misery.

Your living is determined not so much by what life brings to you as by the attitude you bring to life; not so much by what happens to you as by the way your mind looks at what happens.

—Kahlil Gibran

A Stroke's Silver Lining

In 1996, at age thirty-seven, Dr. Jill Bolte Taylor, a Harvard-trained neuroanatomist, suffered a severe stroke. Upon waking one morning, she felt disoriented and began to notice a sensitivity to sound and body sensations, among other symptoms. While showering, she noticed her hands appeared to look like claws, her body was rigid, and the slightest noises became extreme to her. It took Dr. Taylor about four hours to recognize she had had a stroke that affected the left hemisphere of her brain. When her right arm became paralyzed, she knew for sure it was a major stroke. Going into her home office, she tried to recognize her office number on her business card, but her reasoning and language skills were not there. When she finally managed to call her office, she was unable to form words. Fortunately, her associate answered the phone, recognized her voice and, knowing something was not right, called 911. Upon entering Massachusetts General Hospital, Dr. Taylor had no understanding of whom the people were who asked her to sign some papers. During her hospital stay the medical staff appeared distant and unconcerned about her or her condition. A woman she knew in the professional field, whom she dubbed "The Queen of Neurology," entered her room with an entourage of medical students. Dr. Taylor felt safe around this person because she sensed familiarity and respect coming from her, though she did not know her. When her mother, Gigi, arrived, Dr. Taylor had no idea who she was, or for that matter, what a mother was. Gigi crawled into bed with her daughter and held her.

All I knew was this loving, kind, spirit came in, wrapped herself around me and just took ownership of loving me—and that was the new beginning.

—Dr. Jill Bolte Taylor
My Stroke of Insight

After five days, Dr. Taylor went home, where her mother took care of her. Two and a half weeks later, she underwent surgery to remove a tumor from the left hemisphere of her brain. It took eight years for her to completely recover from the stroke. She had to relearn language and left-brain activities, which had virtually disappeared from her memory. Dr. Taylor says it was like a rebirth. On the one hand, her right brain, which holds the feelings, intuitive, and creative parts, was amped up. Disconnected from ego and reasoning, she felt this incredible presence of peace and joy, even though she couldn't speak or understand what was going on around her. On the other hand, her right brain was demonstrating a state of peace and nirvana.

Today, Dr. Taylor has an attitude of gratitude and is able to filter out thoughts from her left brain that do not contribute to her mental health and wholeness. While her long recovery was clearly difficult, in the process she came to believe that we as a species are 99 percent identical, thus making us interconnected beings. Essentially, she realized there is really no separation between us. The left brain has the ability to analyze, feel a sense of ego, reason, use vocabulary, and identify functions. Dr. Taylor says that through this life-altering experience, she has been capable of altering the circuitry that runs through her brain cells, whether conscious or subconscious, to create new rules.

Dr. Taylor is passionately involved as a national spokesperson for the mentally ill and supports postmortem studies on people with schizophrenia and bipolar disorders. She also lends her talent as a musician and travels the country as the Singing Scientist. In 2009, *Time Magazine* awarded Dr. Taylor as one of the "100 Most Influential People in the World." She has also been featured on Oprah's Super Soul Series webcast as well as in interviews with Dr. Oz and Oprah Winfrey.

After listening to Dr. Taylor's story, I have a greater understanding and compassion for my mother, who I'm fairly certain had the ability to observe, but not to communicate. When my mother suffered a stroke at fifty-three, I was living in Florida. I remember trying to comprehend what she was saying to me over the phone as her stroke had impaired her speech. This made her difficult to understand. I could sense her fear and how distraught she sounded, so I kept telling her I loved her and would travel up north to be with her. Sadly, while I was on the trip there, my mother died. How difficult it must have been for her to want to be understood, but not be able to speak clearly to me. My mother always had a controlling personality, and this time she was not able to control what was happening to her body or her mind.

All that we are is the result of what we have thought. If a man speaks or acts with an evil thought, pain follows him. If a man speaks or acts with a pure thought, happiness follows him, like a shadow that never leaves him.

—Buddha

Mind Over Matter

Several years ago, I was asked to donate time to help a group of young people prepare for a Special Olympics swim meet. I felt that I was in a sea of carefree adults in a childlike mind who were so enthusiastic about achieving their goal of swimming from one end of the pool to the other. I was able to communicate with them by getting close, focusing on their faces, and praising them. After our practice sessions, we took the group to the indoor hot tub where they could get warm before heading to the locker room to shower and change. One day, while entering the tubs, another small group of adults seemed to become very uncomfortable with our group, and immediately got out of the pool. Even though it didn't seem to impact our group, it seemed similar to the cold manner of the hospital staff tending to Dr. Taylor. When we treat one another with open respect, kindness, and caring, we all benefit.

In the late 1990s, I was living in a small mountain community in the southwest corner of Colorado. I visited with a German scientist, Adolph Zielinski, who had come to town to try to help a friend of mine who was suffering from a brain tumor. Dr. Zielinski had worked closely with several Russian scientists to decipher and study the brain, much like Dr. Taylor, before and after her stroke. He had traveled around the world using certain right- and left-brain techniques to help stimulate the deeper realms of the brain and activate four stages of brain waves: beta (waking stage), alpha (meditative, daydreaming), theta (creativity, dreams), delta (deep sleep, out of body experiences). During his stay, I was introduced to the various brain waves through a series of sounds of various frequencies that I listened to with a headset. The session lasted an hour. I believe that the frequencies heightened the portion of my brain that stimulated the taste buds. One of the first things I noticed afterward was how food tasted to me. It was as though I had never experienced these tastes before, and they were wonderful. All my senses seemed to be heightened, and a feeling of euphoria surrounded me. I could still think and reason, but the left side of the brain seemed less in command.

A few days after Dr. Zielinski left, I awoke one morning feeling different in my head. I saw rapid pictures as though I was watching a movie in fast forward. I thought, "How strange," and began to feel that the brainwave session was producing some differences in my brain. I was wondering if I could drive to my office. Everything else seemed normal, so I decided it was safe for me to operate my vehicle. Once at my office, I realized my focus and my left-brain activities weren't stimulated. The fast forward images had continued. I left the office and stayed home for two days observing this phenomenon and having a joyful time. On the third day, when I awoke, something was different. The images had faded, my euphoria had diminished, and I felt once again like my original self. It made me sad—I wished I could have maintained the feelings that had given me such a beautiful experience.

Perhaps we can achieve a visceral experience each day of our lives by applying various principles in our own lives, including integrating gratitude and wholeness toward ourselves and others by recognizing that we are all powerful interconnected beings that truly wish to be appreciated and loved.

Scientific Findings

Dr. Bruce Lipton is a passionate scientist. He's devoted his life to understanding human biology and behavior. He received his PhD from the University of Virginia at Charlottesville, and then went on to the University of Wisconsin School of Medicine, where he was an associate professor of anatomy.

In Bruce Lipton's book, *The Biology of Belief*, scientific findings merge with a convergence of the body-mind-spirit trinity to empower our thoughts, beliefs, and attitudes into our daily lives. We are living in a world filled with chaotic energy which affects our path to peace-filled living. Bruce Lipton's scientific studies have shown that our childhood beliefs and programmed perceptions (usually at seven years of age) can be radically shifted and help to rewrite our genetic coding. The conscious mind is our creative mind, the subconscious is our habitual mind which is habitually resistant to change. Neuroscience indicates that our subconscious controls 95 percent of our lives. In the case of my sister and her prognosis of bladder and brain cancer, Dr. Lipton clarifies, "what that means is that your mind will adjust the body's biology and behavior to fit with your beliefs. If you've been told you'll die in six months and your mind believes it, you most likely will die in six months. That's called the nocebo effect, the result of a negative thought, which is the opposite of the placebo effect, where healing is mediated by a positive thought" (Lipton, 2005). My sister tearfully told me six months before her passing that if she didn't have chemo or radiation, she would die. Bruce Lipton states that "Through processes such as hypnosis, subliminal tapes, the religious use of affirmations, Buddhist mindfulness, or a series of reprogramming modalities collectively referred to as energy psychology, such as PSYCH-K, Emotional Self-Management (ESM), Eye Movement Desensitization and Reprocessing (EMDR), and Emotional Freedom Techniques (EFT), among many other new techniques, we can rewrite those destructive programs that occupy our subconscious field." (Lipton, 2005).

His research is in tune with *The Power of Positive Thinking* and *The Laws of Attraction.* Bruce Lipton's new science of cellular biology can inspire us personally and professionally.

I have learned to think of everything I see as having an energetic template that makes it appear as it does in the physical. When I want to change something in my life, I start with changing my energy. I do that by changing my belief about it and the emotions that I associate with it. It might sound crazy, but ... that is what the Law of Attraction is all about.

—Bruce Lipton, PhD

Yale School of Public Health

According to DavidWolfe.com, individuals who have a negative attitude toward aging have a more likely chance of developing dementia and Alzheimer's according to this study. The Baltimore Longitudinal Study on Aging is the oldest aging study which began in 1958. The study followed 158 people for twenty-five years. At the average age of sixty-eight, these people who had displayed more negative attitudes on aging also had hippocampal (memory) loss. Stress played a major factor.

De-Stress, Naturally

Cortisol and Stress

Do you have any of the following health challenges: Type 1 and 2 diabetes, muscle loss, heart disease, memory loss, depression, high blood pressure, obesity, or autoimmune disease? If so, the stress hormone, cortisol, may be affecting your health.

When we're stressed, suffer physical trauma, or put out extreme physical exertion, our cortisol levels increase to help maintain homeostasis. However, our cortisol levels also increase as we age and may stay high for longer periods of time, which can be extremely toxic. Brain cells are sensitive to the effects of cortisol; excess cortisol could cause damage to brain cells, compromise the immune system, decrease muscle mass, and shrink organs. When we suffer from unmanaged stress, our thyroid glands are impaired, and adrenals go into overload.

There are some symptoms that occur if our cortisol levels are high.

- You like to eat unhealthy food.
- You do not sleep well.
- You have more fat buildup around your abdomen.
- You have a low sex drive.
- Your immune system is low, and you have illnesses.
- You may experience nausea, heartburn, abdominal cramps, diarrhea, or constipation.
- You may feel depressed.
- You may experience body pain.

I personally have an acute sense of adrenal burnout, and experience symptoms such as extreme agitation. When this happens, I take stock of my emotions and activities, rest more, and am determined to have more fun and relaxation in my life. I also watch what I eat and drink, monitor my thoughts, and remove myself from any stressful and disruptive outside disturbances.

De-stress and Release Disease

Stress is closely linked to many diseases. Studies have shown that stress causes immune systems to become compromised and produce higher levels of interleukin 6, a protein that modulates immune responses. When IL-6 measures in higher concentrations, it can accelerate colds, flu, and other illnesses, as well as contribute to poorer cognitive functioning. Plasma fibrinogen in the bloodstream indicates the presence of inflammation. When we are under stress, we produce higher levels of this chemical, which may compromise heart health. Happy people produce lower levels of plasma fibrinogen. This is another reason to smile.

In the past decade, a worldwide increase in depression has led to a rise in the use of antidepressants globally. By the year 2020, depression may be considered the number two cause of disease worldwide, according to the World Health Organization. Would you care to venture a guess as to how many people are on antidepressants in the United States? Try 18.8 million.

Prozac, Zoloft, and Paxil are just a few antidepressants in the marketplace. A couple members of my family have taken them at one time or another. I understand they can be useful for some people. My choice so far is to seek other ways to achieve peace and happiness without a doctor's prescription. If you are considering or have been taking antidepressants, ask your pharmacist and doctor what kind of side effects there may be. Education is your best resource.

Mind-Enhancing Transmitters

Depression has a lot to do with nutrition and mood transmitters. For instance, if we lack energy mentally and physically, we may turn to coffee or sugar as temporary stimulants. Instead of coffee or sugar, one might consider 5-Hydroxytryptophan (5-HTP), an amino acid which enhances serotonin levels in the brain. Another option is L-Tryptophan, an amino acid that also is a neurotransmitter for our brain, taken before bed. In only one month, you may notice a shift in your feelings—all for the better. You may feel more positive, easygoing, and better able to handle stress.

L-Tryptophan is found in high-protein foods such as turkey, pork, beef, chicken, eggs, and dairy products. Many vegetarians produce lower-than-normal levels of serotonin, so in these cases supplementing with L-Tryptophan can be a good idea. Consult with your practitioner before taking supplements.

Endorphins

The body produces three categories of endorphins: beta (usually released in the pituitary gland), enkephalins, and dynorphins (Dyn), which make up the class of opioid peptides associated with the nervous system. Some food sources that produce endorphins include chocolate and spicy chili peppers. Endorphins reduce pain in the body, act as an appetite modulator, release sex hormones, and create feelings of euphoria like “runner’s high.” Endorphins also enhance the immune system and help delay the aging process. Furthermore, they can play a crucial role in helping drug and alcohol abusers overcome their addictions. When our endorphins are low, we may avoid intimacy or confrontation, handle our emotions in an unhealthy manner, and/or turn to substances such as drugs, alcohol, and food. Stimulating the production of endorphins through exercise can help the addictions to subside.

Endorphins are naturally produced by a wide range of activities like hearty laughter, meditation and/or deep breathing, acupuncture, or chiropractic treatments. Tyrosine is an amino acid that helps increase the production of endorphins in the body. It’s considered a natural antidepressant, assisting in producing thyroid hormones, which is a basic factor in our adrenals. Tyrosine is considered one of our most pleasure-promoting chemicals. The molecular structure of tyrosine is very similar to morphine but with different chemical properties. Tyrosine, which is produced in the body from phenylalanine, is found in soy products, chicken, turkey, fish, peanuts, almonds, avocados, bananas, milk, cheese, yogurt, cottage cheese, lima beans, pumpkin seeds, and sesame seeds.

Phenylalanine is also very similar to tyrosine in that it produces euphoria and helps subdue pain. D-phenylalanine is a very potent endorphin. GABA (gamma aminobutyric acid) is both an amino acid and a neurotransmitter. GABA helps alleviate stress and acts as a natural Valium.

Brain Food from the Sea

In a current study at Rush University Medical Center in Chicago, Dr. Martha Clare Morris has followed 3,718 people sixty-five and older for six years. Participants ate fish high in omega-3 fatty acids, which included DHA (docosahexaenoic acid), a fatty acid found in the meat of cold-water fish, including mackerel, herring, tuna, halibut, salmon, cod liver, whale blubber, and seal blubber. DHA is responsible for early brain development. Those over sixty-five who ate fish twice or more a week showed their rate of cognitive decline reduced 10 to 13 percent per year. Eating deep-sea fish like salmon, cod, or halibut at least once a week reduced their mental aging by as much as three years.

Nutrition—Exercise and Sleep for Our Brain

Diet, exercise, and sleep are vital components in reducing brain aging. Nutrition plays an important role in keeping our brain smart. Breakfast that supplies protein, not sugar, gives the brain a jump start. Eggs are rich in acetylcholine, a neurotransmitter. Low levels of this have been linked to patients with Alzheimer's. Salads are packed with antioxidants to help prevent free radicals from forming and provide better cognitive skills. Yogurt contains tyrosine, an amino acid, which helps our memory and alertness. Fruits, in particular blueberries and strawberries, help improve our memory, coordination, and concentration. Eating healthy foods promotes our overall well-being.

Exercising boosts our cognitive abilities. It may be as simple as taking a walk several times a week. Our brain can grow new cells, and exercising helps achieve this. Yoga has many different movements which are forward and backward. Backward bends seem to boost the mental state, which could explain why I feel elated after class. A good night's sleep recharges our brain cells. There may be moments during our sleep in which we can create new thought and wake up with creative new ideas in our head. In this section there is more description on the benefits of a good night's sleep.

Research on Brain and Immune System

The University of Virginia School of Medicine has discovered vessels between the brain and the immune system. This discovery could help people with Alzheimer's, autism, and multiple sclerosis.

Kevin Lee, PhD, chair of the UVA Department of Neuroscience states, "The first time these guys showed me the basic result, I just said one sentence: 'They'll have to change the textbooks.' There has never been a lymphatic system for the central nervous system, and it was very clear from that first singular observation—and they've done many studies since then to bolster the finding—that it will fundamentally change the way people look at the central nervous system's relationship with the immune system" (Newsroom, 2015).

Kipping believes that the protein chunks that accumulate in the brain had no vessels available to remove them (Science News, 2015).

Brain and Immunity

"Instead of asking, 'How do we study the immune response of the brain?' 'Why do multiple sclerosis patients have the immune attacks?' now we can approach this mechanistically. Because the brain is like every other tissue connected to the peripheral immune system through meningeal lymphatic vessels," said Jonathan Kipnis, PhD, professor in the UVA Department of Neuroscience and director of UVA's Center for Brain Immunology and Glia (BIG). "It changes entirely the way we perceive the neuro-immune interaction. We always perceived it before as something esoteric that can't be studied. But now we can ask mechanistic questions."

"We believe that for every neurological disease that has an immune component to it, these vessels may play a major role," Kipnis said. "Hard to imagine that these vessels would not be involved in a [neurological] disease with an immune component."

Brain Injuries

Could there be a link among people who suffer brain damage from blood hemorrhages, automobile accidents, and falls? Dr. Sandra Magnoni of the Ospedale Maggiore Policlinico Trauma Center in Milan, Italy inserted a catheter into eighteen patients' brains for three to seven days to observe the beta-amyloid levels (an Alzheimer's-related protein). The beta-amyloid measurements may indicate how well the cells are communicating with each other. In

Alzheimer's patients, a sticky gooey form bathes the brain rather than a fluid. Scientists have not yet connected the purpose of the beta-amyloid or what triggers the plaque formations within the brain. A person with brain injuries may develop dementia later in life. If continued studies and research can show a link between brain damage and increased beta-amyloid connection, it may help to lower the risk of Alzheimer's disease.

Preventing Alzheimer's

Today, five million people suffer from Alzheimer's disease in America. It is the seventh leading cause of death, and it affects one in eight people aged sixty-five and older and one-half of those eighty-five and older. More than twenty-six million people worldwide were estimated to be living with Alzheimer's disease in 2006, according to a study led by researchers at the Johns Hopkins Bloomberg School of Public Health. This figure could grow to 106 million by 2050. In Asia, over 48 percent of Alzheimer cases are currently documented.

Dr. Gary Small Study

Dr. Gary Small is a neuroscientist who, along with the University of California, performed a fourteen-day study of thirty-four adults with average memories and an average age of fifty-three years. They were asked to perform a series of functions, including behavior modification, brisk walks, and physical conditioning, along with stretching and relaxation techniques. They were also put on a memory improvement plan that included exercises such as crossword puzzles and brain teasers. They ate five small meals per day featuring omega-3 fats from fish and olive oil, whole grain carbohydrates, and antioxidants.

At the beginning and end of the fourteen-day trial, the volunteers were given a PET (positron emission tomography) scan that measured activity throughout the brain. Results showed that memory improved while using less brain power. Dr. Small and others state that it is never too late or too early to get started on a healthy lifestyle to improve brain power. *Publishers Weekly* has featured The Alzheimer's Prevention Program in its Top Ten Lifestyle/Health & Fitness category. Dr. Small's book, *The Alzheimer's Prevention Program*, is a must-read for people who are seeking preventive measures for Alzheimer's disease.

Another study by the MacArthur Foundation found that seniors who were physically active maintained a higher level of brain function over a ten-year period dating from the beginning of the study. Also, genetics don't always play a dominant role mentally and physically; regular exercise can outweigh the genetic blueprint. And according to the Mayo Clinic, you may be able to lower your risk of Alzheimer's disease by reducing your risk of heart disease. Many of the same factors that increase your risk of heart disease can also increase your risk of Alzheimer's disease and vascular dementia. Important factors that may be involved include high blood pressure, high blood cholesterol, excess weight, and diabetes.

Queensland Brain Institute (QBI)

A focused therapeutic ultrasound sends harmless u sound waves into the brain tissue. The blood brain barrier is a layer which protects the brain from bacteria. The sound waves gently penetrate this barrier. This stimulates microglial cells (waste removal cells) to clear out the beta-amyloid clumps, which is a critical Alzheimer's condition. According to an article on DavidWolfe.com, when sound waves were tested on mice, there was a 75 percent improvement in brain function. However, the brain of a human is twice the size of a mouse, so continued research will be necessary.

Preventive Suggestions

Older adults who stay mentally active may be at lower risk.

- Staying physically active; walking, exercise program, yoga
- Reading
- Playing cards and board games

- Crossword puzzles
- Staying social
- Eat more fruits and vegetables, high fiber foods, fish, and omega-3-rich oils (Mediterranean diet which is discussed in this book)
- Healthy weight, lower blood pressure

Hope for Alzheimer's

It appears that the longer one lives, the higher the risk of developing Alzheimer's. The disease has been linked to a protein known as beta-amyloid, which collects between nerve cells, thus disrupting brain function and triggering an immune response that destroys the cells. Scientists have been testing viable new drugs, which will give hope to those with low to moderate levels of the disease.

Medical Drugs

Cholinesterase Inhibitors for Early to Moderate Stages

Cholinesterase inhibitors are prescribed to treat symptoms related to memory, thinking, language, judgment, and other thought processes.

- Donepezil (Aricept) is approved to treat all stages of Alzheimer's.
- Rivastigmine (Exelon) is approved to treat mild to moderate Alzheimer's.
- Galantamine (Razadyne) is approved to treat mild to moderate Alzheimer's.

Medication for Moderate to Severe Stages

A second type of medication, memantine (Namenda) is approved by the FDA for treatment of moderate to severe Alzheimer's.

Memantine is prescribed to improve memory, attention, reason, language, and the ability to perform simple tasks.

University of Virginia Study

A 2015 University of Virginia School of Medicine study establishes a direct link of newly discovered vessels which connect to the immune system through the brain.

Kevin Lee, PhD, chair of the UVA Department of Neuroscience, states from the lab study, "The first time these guys showed me the basic result, I just said one sentence: 'They'll have to change the textbooks.' There has never been a lymphatic system for the central nervous system, and it was very clear from that first singular observation—and they've done many studies since then to bolster the finding—that it will fundamentally change the way people look at the central nervous system's relationship with the immune system" (Newsroom, 2015).

According to Jonathan Kipnis, PhD, professor in the UVA Department of Neuroscience and Director of UVA's Center for BIG, "In Alzheimer's, there are accumulations of big protein chunks in the brain," Kipnis said. "We think they may be accumulating in the brain because they're not being efficiently removed by these vessels" (Newsroom, 2015). He noted that the vessels look different with age, so the role they play in aging is another avenue to explore. And there's an enormous array of other neurological diseases, from autism to multiple sclerosis, that must be reconsidered in light of the presence of something science insisted did not exist.

Vitamin E

In 2014, results of a study published in the *Journal of the American Medical Association* showed that individuals with mild to moderate Alzheimer's disease who received high doses of vitamin E had a 19 percent slower rate of functional decline than study volunteers who received a placebo. Functional decline includes problems with daily activities such as shopping, preparing meals, bathing, eating, planning, and traveling. Study participants were followed up for an average of a little more than two years. Participants in the study who received both vitamin E and the FDA-approved Alzheimer's drug memantine did not show the same benefit as participants who received vitamin E alone.

Alzheimer's Association Organization

A United States research study has shown that people who take angiotensin-receptor blockers are 35 to 40 percent less likely to develop Alzheimer's disease. Angiotensin-receptor blockers are drugs that are used to lower blood pressure. In addition to the good news with respect to preventing Alzheimer's disease, the study showed that even if a person already has the illness, starting the angiotensin-receptor blockers would slow the progression of the illness down by 45 percent. Professor Clive Ballard of the Alzheimer's Research Society stated that the study essentially encouraged more investigation into blood pressure lowering drugs as a potential treatment for dementia.

How to Join a Clinical Trial

When it comes to Alzheimer's, buying any time at all is a good idea. Therefore, early detection is a key to slowing the disease, and researchers urge participation in clinical trials. "To take part in a trial is a great gift to society," says William Thies, Vice President of Medical and Scientific Relations for the Alzheimer's Association.

Alzheimer's TrialMatch is seeking individuals for ongoing trial studies, email: trialmatch@alz.org or call 800.272.3900.

To find out more about clinical trials and studies in your area refer to the reference section at the back of this book.

A Daughter's Approach to Alzheimer's Disease

My friend Sally traveled to Vermont to visit her parents, when they were in their nineties. Her dad lived at home and her mom had been in a care facility for the last three years because it became increasingly difficult for her dad to watch over her, though he traveled a few short miles each day to visit and have dinner with her. When my friend was there, she asked her mom (who did not recognize her daughter anymore) if she would like to let her husband know she is tired and wishes to leave her body. Sally said her mom's face lit up and she nodded. So Sally took the big step in talking to her dad about this incident. Her father went to see her mother but would not discuss any of the sharing that Sally and her mom had.

Sally felt that if her dad would tell her mother that it is OK for her to leave her body, she would. Sally felt her dad was holding on to his wife emotionally, and that she sensed this. Her condition continued to deteriorate, and she rarely went outside. Sally realized that she needed to leave this heartbreaking situation in the hands of her father. Later, her father's deteriorating health led to the decision for her father to move into the same facility that his wife was in. He had major diabetes and had heart bypass surgery ten years before. Sally's mother had moved from the Alzheimer's floor to the general ailment section of the care facility. There, they spent days together eating meals and seeing each other. Sally's dad learned to accept help easier since he didn't live in his own home or drive his car any longer.

Sally's loving story reminded me of Nicholas Sparks's book, *The Notebook*, in which two people married and lived devotedly for many years. The wife developed Alzheimer's and didn't recognize her family or husband except for brief moments. Her husband moved into the same facility, where they passed away serenely in each other's arms. There are various stories which contain different dynamics around family members who have Alzheimer's.

How do we care for our loved ones and how can we afford to have them in an extended care facility? Can we care for them in their home or have them move into ours? The Alzheimer's Foundation of America is an excellent resource to help guide people through the process and help create a better quality of life.

Prevent Aging

Telomeres are protective caps on each end of our chromosomes. When our cells divide, the telomeres shorten. Eventually they reach a critical point, and the cell stops dividing and dies. Diseases such as heart disease, cancer, diabetes, and Alzheimer's have all been linked to shortened telomeres. Elizabeth H. Blackburn, PhD, received the 2009 Nobel Peace Prize in telomere research. Elissa Epel, a University of California researcher, has stated that there is a strong mind-cell connection to the length of our telomeres. When we are stressed, living in the past or the future, multitasking and ruminating, this affects the length of our telomeres. A University of California study was done having people meditating in the Colorado mountains for three months. The results showed they slowed their aging process compared to people who were in the control group.

Prevention

- Meditating
- Staying in the present moment
- Exercise
- Vitamins B12, C, and D, and multivitamin
- Magnesium
- Antioxidant supplement
- Green tea
- Healthy weight

- Relaxation techniques
- Breathing exercises
- Adding omega-3 foods
- Abstain from smoking and alcohol.

Cultivating a Healthy Mind and Brain

I offer the following suggestions as catalysts for your continuing quest for improved immunity and vitality.

I. Be Grateful—Develop an Attitude of Gratitude

When there is something that may not be going well, rather than focusing on what is wrong and how you can fix it, ask yourself, "What do I have in my life right now to be grateful for?" This simple exercise doesn't make problems go away but rather makes them less important for the moment. Focusing on gratitude can help you find a solution to the current situation, as you are better able to cope with difficulties by addressing them with a gracious and grateful nature.

- Rather than concentrating on what you don't have, give thanks for each day by focusing on the amazing things in your life.
- Make a list of people and things in your life you are grateful for.
- Greet people with a smile or do something kind for another.
- Don't allow pressures in your life to let you forget to be grateful.

II. Be Creative—Express Yourself in Artful Ways

We are never too old to create. It could be painting a sunset, throwing a piece of pottery on the wheel, touring an art museum, looking at beautiful architecture or just allowing your imagination to run wild. Remember as children we eagerly dove into finger painting, coloring, drawing, or making clay objects. I have taken classes in both stained glass and weaving; they were challenging as well as extremely rewarding. I have also studied pottery and look forward to making a clay piece someday soon. Recently I have been taking my camera with me to capture various images—creative activities, all.

- Boost your intuitive nature by taking an art class.
- Read books.
- Write a story.
- Visit an art museum or exhibit.
- Take photographs of images that inspire you.
- Create a beautiful space in your home or garden.

III. Be Active—Get Out and Move

Active bodies keep our minds sharp and create more flexibility in our lives. Sitting around too much drags us down and compromises our health. You don't have to become a professional athlete. I weave in and out of yoga and Pilates classes. Each day I do something to keep my heart pumping and my body strong, knowing that I am taking care of myself through exercise and a healthy diet.

- Take walks or bike whenever you can and leave your car at home.
- Join a Pilates, yoga, or weight training class and have fun.
- Strive to do things that you thought you could not do.
- Stretch your body and breathe deeply during the day.
- Take up an outdoor sport—learn how to ski, swim or even sail.

IV. Be Inspired

Inspiration means to be *in spirit* and comes from being fully present and full of vitality each day. We may be inspired by looking at the starlit night or hearing a beautiful symphony. Often when I am working on a book project, I let my imagination take hold. I may read a passage that inspires or witness a wondrous sunset; listen to beautiful music or go for a swim. Inspiration keeps us bursting open and makes us feel more alive. It is an internal feeling that touches each of us in unique ways. Live expressively by filling your home with flowers, music, and anything that inspires you. Accept and expect all that is good in life, both inside and out, and discover your unique role in life—what brings you passion and enthusiasm?

- Read inspiring books.
- Leap into action by doing something worthwhile for your community or an organization.
- Turn off the television, radio, and other distractions, and sit quietly and listen to that still voice within.
- Inspire others by sharing your own purpose through ideas and abilities.
- Be true to yourself and your ideals.

V. Connect with Nature

As a child I relished living outdoors in the summertime. I would canoe miles of lakes or river inlets hearing the bottom of my boat go swoosh over the water lilies while observing the ambitious beavers piling wood to build their homes. I swam every day, sometimes for miles across the lake or went hiking on a trail or up a mountain. Sometimes I found myself simply lying in a field of wildflowers while the honeybees drank nectar. One period of my life, I volunteered at the Audubon Preserve along the shores of Lake Michigan. Nature has always given me peace of mind and a great appreciation for life.

- Get out in nature and witness the natural beauty and stillness around you.
- Live around nature if at all possible.
- If you live in the city, visit a park or arboretum.
- Sign up for nature hikes and programs.
- Listen to the sounds of nature.

Climb the mountains and get their good tidings. Nature's peace will flow into you as sunshine flows into trees. The winds will blow their own freshness into you, and the storms their energy, while cares will drop off like autumn leaves.

—John Muir

VI. Be Selfish—Treat and Pamper Yourself

Being selfish is a difficult thing for many of us to aspire to. And yet it is important for us to learn how to be kinder to ourselves. I raised five children and had very little time to do things for myself that didn't involve the family. I disciplined myself to make time for just me. Sometimes I was able to squeeze in an hour away. Sometimes it was as simple as a walk or a lunch with a friend. In the long run it made me a more tolerant and happier mother and wife. Serve yourself. You deserve it.

- Schedule a day at a spa for a massage and facial.
- Have lunch with a friend.
- Have your family do the chores for a day.
- See a play or listen to a concert.
- Soak in a long bath and don't forget to lock the door.

Benefits of Meditation

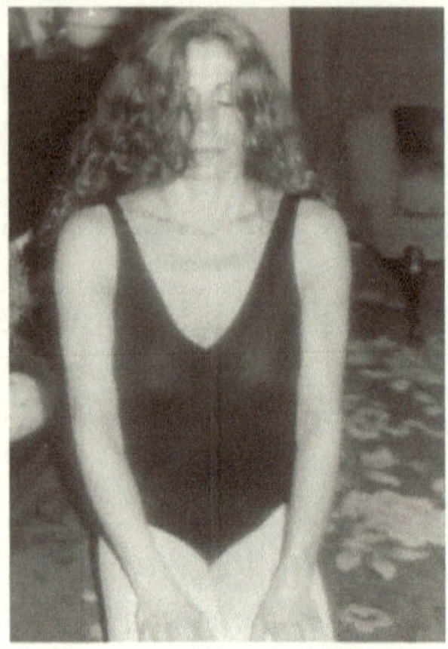

Author meditating in her thirties.

- Meditation increases the thickness of the cerebral cortex—an area of the brain associated with sensory and attention processes.
- Meditation can bring calmness, peace, and a joyful expression.
- Meditation can help reduce stress and pain.
- Meditation helps with respiratory and cardiovascular functions.
- Meditation reduces stress, improves the immune system, and lowers blood pressure.
- Take supplements: tyrosine, phenylalanine, and GABA, which help to alleviate stress.
- Learn breathing techniques. Close your eyes—breathe normally through your nose—be aware of breathing in and out. Expand belly as you inhale, belly in as you exhale. Do a count of four for each in and out.

VII. Be Mellow

Let's face it. We live in a complicated and stressful world. You may live in a big city and commute to work, or you may currently be out of work. There may be an illness or other challenge within your family. You may live alone and find your life lonely and uninspiring. There are ways to counter stress, each person copes with stress in their own way. You may internalize it and keep it bottled up inside. You may become extremely agitated and angry. You may drink, eat unhealthy foods, take drugs or smoke too much. You may get panic attacks or make yourself ill. The cortisol level in our body increases as we age, affecting our brain cells and immune system. Stress also creates higher levels of cortisol, which helps to create the stubborn fat in the stomach that we can't seem to lose no matter what we do. You can counter stress with the following suggestions.

- Herbs (check with your practitioner if on a prescribed medicine); Serenity® by Gaia Herbs, usually found in a health store or online, contains Kava Kava and other herbs to steady the nerves.

- Refer to the supplement section herein, which addresses ways you can alleviate stress, including tyrosine, phenylalanine, and GABA.

VIII. Be Rested—How to Have a Good Night's Sleep

My seventy-five-year-old grandmother who had diabetes mellitus type 2 would often read a book in the middle of the night. One time I asked her why. Her response was simply, "At my age, I can't afford to sleep." I understood her intentions and yet, a good night's sleep is important for our well-being. Dr. Eve Van Cauter at the University of Chicago found that chronic sleep deprivation—defined as six and a half hours or less of sleep per night—has the same effect on insulin resistance as aging. Along with poor diet, a sedentary lifestyle, aging and chronic stress, lack of sleep is a risk factor for type 2 diabetes.

I sleep eight to nine hours each night and rise early in the morning. There are times I take a thirty-minute cat nap during the middle part of the day, with my kitty, of course. My sister was the opposite. She often stayed up until one a.m. and still got up early to go to work.

- Avoid bedtime snacks, particularly grains, sugar, caffeine, liquor, high fat or spicy meals; these will raise blood sugar levels, stimulate digestion, and make sleep difficult; later, when blood sugar levels drop too low (hypoglycemia), you might wake up and not be able to fall back asleep.

- Combining B vitamins with calcium and magnesium can calm your nervous system; beans, turkey, chicken, nuts, eggs, and dairy contain high levels of B vitamins.

- Eat foods that enhance serotonin levels (such as salmon, hummus, and baked tempeh) a few hours before bedtime; this helps to balance our sugar levels and provide for a more restful sleep.

- Do not watch television or work in bed; read spiritual or inspirational literature for a few minutes before bed and avoid dramatic novels or distressing reading material; once in bed, close your eyes and simply feel your body—and wherever you notice tension, consciously relax that area—then, simply pay attention to your slow, easy breathing until you fall asleep.

- Go to bed as early as possible; prior to the invention of electricity, people went to bed shortly after sundown, as most animals do, which is what nature intended for humans as well. The body systems, particularly the adrenal glands, do a majority of their recovering during the hours of eleven p.m. and one a.m. In addition, the gallbladder dumps toxins during this time; if you are awake, those toxins back up into the liver—which then secondarily back up into your entire system, causing further disruption to your health.

- Aim to be in your bed with the lights out between 9:30 and 10:30 p.m.; if you are not used to getting to bed this early, move your bedtime up by thirty minutes every week until you are in bed by 10:30; for example, if you usually watch television until midnight, try turning off the TV at 11:30 for a week; then aim for thirty minutes earlier; and finally to bed at 10:30 p.m.

- Stay away from alcohol; although alcohol makes you drowsy at first, its effect is short-lived, and you often wake up after a few hours. Alcohol will also prevent you from falling into the deeper stages of sleep, when the body does most of its healing.

- Avoid foods to which you may be sensitive; this is particularly true for dairy and wheat products, because they have been shown to cause sleep apnea, gastrointestinal upset, excess congestion, and gas, among other things.

- Try to reduce or avoid as many drugs as possible; many medications, both prescription and over the counter, may affect sleep.

- Create a peaceful, dark bedroom.

- There are a variety of herbs for a sound sleep; some herbal supplement suggestions are Melatonin, Serotonin, Lavender, Chamomile, Hops, and Valerian; drink a nighttime herbal tea or soak in an herbal bath.

Consult with your practitioner if you are having difficulty sleeping and wish to substitute a more natural approach than prescription medicine.

IV. Be Healthy and Happy

By starting with this book, I hope you have been inspired to become healthier. Being healthy and happy encompasses the food we eat, our daily attitudes, and the environment where we live, which includes our community of family and friends. We can choose to change our diet, exercise more or be of service to another who may need help.

I have told Dr. Norman Cousin's story of his illness and his empowering decisions to engage in laughter and heal his medical condition. Anything is possible. Choose happiness each day. It may be as simple as eating a scrumptious juicy apple just picked from a tree. It could be lying in a hammock with one of your grandchildren or witnessing a splendid rainbow after a misty rain. True happiness comes from deep within us.

- Smile every day.
- Laugh often.
- Eat fresh, healthy foods.
- Spend time with family or friends.
- Give thanks for your life each day.
- Help someone in need.

Each morning when I open my eyes I say to myself: I, not events, have the power to make me happy or unhappy today. I can choose which it shall be. Yesterday is dead, tomorrow hasn't arrived yet. I have just one day, today, and I'm going to be happy in it.

—Groucho Marx

Be Smart—Our Thoughts and Our Choices

Peaceful sleep and following current mind research can help fight the effects of the diseases associated with aging. We can also change our mind about life situations. A book and video called *The Secret* made its debut in 2006. It has become a national bestseller and was featured on *The Oprah Winfrey Show*. The gist of the material is the law of attraction, which states that what we believe, we draw into our lives and that becomes our reality. We do not live in a perfect world. But how we react and respond to our earthly experiences molds our identity along with our state of health, peace of mind and consciousness. Who we are evolves from the world we create with our choice of experiences and associations.

If you feel overwhelmed with any situation, put it aside and make a list of all the people and experiences that you are grateful for at this moment in your life. You will see your perspective shift toward a more positive attitude.

Beliefs have the power to create and the power to destroy. Human beings have the awesome ability to take any experience of their lives and create a meaning that disempowers them or one that can literally save their lives.

—Anthony Robbins

Step 2

Your Body: The Vehicle That Lasts a Lifetime

Physical fitness is not only one of the most important keys to a healthy body, but also the basis of dynamic and creative intellectual activity.

—John F. Kennedy

How Our Body Image Reflects Wholeness

I have lived my entire life knowing the importance of keeping my body strong, stretched, and moving. While my siblings and I were growing up in the forties and fifties we were as active as any other children. We were rarely inside; we rode our bikes to school, played all kinds of sports, and went to summer camp. Even though my grandparents, parents, aunts, and uncles were not physically active people (and were not slim, either), my mother had the foresight to send us to camp until we were seventeen, and then my sister and I were tennis instructors at a camp on Lake Champlain in Vermont. My sister had polio before the Salk vaccine came out, so my brother and I were sent away from home until she recovered (her spine gave her difficulty throughout her lifetime). My brother was a football player in high school and college, and being a tall and large-muscled person, his weight escalated at times to 260 pounds. He broke his hip in his early sixties while on his bike. It was a painful journey back and to this day one leg is slightly shorter than the other. He recently retired and has high hopes of getting back to an exercise program.

After I married, my family often went camping and my husband and I played doubles in tennis matches. I had horses, skied, hiked, swam, and basically continued being physically active. The only time my weight ballooned was when I was in high school. I have had small weight gains through the years but never more than a ten-to-fifteen-pound increase. My sister had an active metabolism so whatever she ate was burned off. As an adult she never prepared meals at home for herself, especially after her divorce. I was flabbergasted when I tried to cook for her when she had cancer. Her dishwasher was never used, her garbage disposal had been broken for two years, and her cooking pots were brand new. She would order takeout food or eat at restaurants. When she was in chemotherapy, I would make her breakfast and we would sit at her dining room table, something she never did. She told me she never ate breakfast at home; instead, she would grab a chocolate bar on the way to her office. She worked out at a local gym; however, she seemed off balance when it came to other areas of her life.

Today, skinny models project a perfect Barbie-like figure. At the other end of the spectrum, children and teenagers are becoming more obese, at least in part because schools have eliminated or cut back on gym classes. People sit in front of computer and television screens more frequently, both at home and on the job. Sixty percent of Americans are now classed as overweight. We are flooded with commercials for weight loss plans and diet pills galore. If we have poor self-esteem it is reflected in drinking, eating, drugs, and abusive behavior. The key is to get help and demonstrate a more kind and positive nature toward ourselves. Then we can begin to foster better health naturally, through improved foods, exercise, and mental balance.

Six Physical Stages of a Woman's Life

This section talks about a multitude of ways to get and stay fit in one's lifetime. It's all up to us to be motivated to be and stay healthy. For some, it may be more challenging if you haven't been moving and exercising for a while. Be kind to yourself and take steps to do something each day; walk with friends, attend an easy yoga class, go out dancing with someone special, join a gym nearby and talk to a trainer about a program you can start with. The following stages of our lives provide a blueprint for our bodies and how they change. I hope you find them very informative and useful. I wish to credit this information to Joanna Soh (www.joannasoh.com). She has amazing exercises on her site as well as on Facebook. Check out her healthy food recipes as well!

The Twenties

Active woman

- Weight 45-65 kgs (95-143 lb.).
- Body fat: 18-22%.
- Excellent metabolism, strength, stamina, and flexibility.

Sedentary woman

- 50 to 65 kgs (110-143 lb.).
- Body fat: 23-30%.
- Metabolism low, body fat high, muscle mass low.

The Thirties

Active woman

- Body fat: 20-24%.
- Metabolic rate lower, body fat higher (can be improved with exercise).

Sedentary woman

- Body fat: 24-32%.
- Loses 3-5% muscle mass per decade (after 30).
- Metabolism low, increased fat in tummy, hips, and thighs.
- Cardiovascular and metabolic diseases.
- Lack of strength and energy.

- Reduce calories by 150-200 a day.
- Losing weight becomes increasingly more difficult.

The Forties

Active woman

- Body fat: 23-27%.
- Muscle loss due to increase in body fat.
- Strength and stamina (light drop).
- Lifting weights and running help build strong bones.

Sedentary woman

- Body fat: 28-34%.
- Rapid weight gain.
- Heavier, weaker, slower, and stiffer.
- Lose 1-1½ inches in height.
- Decrease in muscle mass and bone density.
- May lead to osteoporosis.
- Hormonal changes.
- Shift to bigger meals early in day; lighter meals in evening.

The Fifties

Active woman

- Body fat: 27-31%.
- Avoid joints wear and tear with lower impact exercise—swimming, cycling, or yoga.
- Loss of skin elasticity.

Sedentary woman

- Body fat: 33-37%.
- Weight: 70-100 kgs (154-200 lb.).
- High blood pressure and cholesterol.
- Lower back pain.
- Sagging breasts and tummy.
- Energy: 30% less than in 20s.
- Eat 4-5 smaller meals.

The Sixties

Active woman

- Body fat: 28-31%.
- Healthy appetite and healthy weight.
- Menopause; bones strong because of years of strength training.
- Skin—good condition.

Sedentary woman

- Body fat: 34-38%.
- Two or three inches shorter in height.
- Lose appetite and appear frail.
- Breasts sag and hips and waist widen.
- 10-15% weaker heart.
- Skin dry.
- Decrease in food intake can lower protein in your muscles

and bone mass.

The Seventies

Active woman

- Body fat: 31-34%.
- Carry on daily routines easily.
- Strong body, heart, and attitude.
- Look and feel twenty years younger.
- Wrinkles and dry skin because of loss of oils after menopause.

Sedentary woman

- Body fat: + 38%.
- Slow movements.
- Constantly in pain, discomfort, and exhausted very easily.
- High blood pressure.
- Brittle bones, high cholesterol levels.
- Medications.
- Very dry skin, lots of wrinkles, and sadness.

Exercise and Health: The Benefits

A. Boost Your Metabolism

Our metabolism converts food and stored fat into energy. As we age, our metabolism slows, but exercise can speed it up. Exercise is crucial to a healthy life, especially in our later years.

Research shows that increased daily activity plus a toned physique can help accelerate the body's metabolism. Lean muscle mass makes your metabolism work faster and stronger. Exercising just thirty minutes a day increases muscle mass which helps to keep the metabolic rate higher at any age. Exercise and normal daily activities also aid in burning more calories due to the cells' increased labor. You can also boost your metabolism by eating smaller quantities of food throughout the day rather than three large meals. Avoid trans fats, drink more purified water, and choose whole grain and fresh foods. We'll discuss all of this in detail further in the book.

Basal Metabolic Rate

An important measurement of metabolism is the basal metabolic rate (BMR). The BMR is the amount of energy expended to support basic bodily functions such as your heartbeat, breathing, walking, sleeping, and brain activity. Men typically have a 10 to 15 percent faster BMR than women. The resting metabolic rate, which is closely related to the BMR, makes up 50 to 75 percent of our daily caloric expenditure and depends on the size of our bodies.

B. Prevent Joint Pain and Arthritis

My mother had severe rheumatoid arthritis, but not once did her doctors suggest an exercise program for fear that movement would put more stress on her swollen joints. Today, it is known that exercise can help alleviate pain in the knees and hips. Along with more traditional care, current views on the management of arthritis include aerobic exercise and resistance training to strengthen muscles around joints and take the pressure off the joints themselves. Stretching keeps the body flexible, while aerobic exercise can help with weight control, thereby relieving the strain on joints.

C. Prevent Osteoporosis

Bone loss can in some cases be reversed and bone health can be maintained through exercise, including walking and hiking, weight training, stretching, and yoga at least thirty minutes to an hour five days a week. You will be rewarded with more flexibility and fewer injuries and falls. Exercise assists in developing muscle strength and building bones. Discuss with your doctor a unique exercise program for your body. If you have developed fractures, consult with your practitioner about a safe way to exercise.

Heart Rate

To gain the most from your cardio exercise regimen, first determine your target maximum working heart rate by deducting your age from 220. Once you have that number, during the first few weeks of your exercise program, aim at the lowest part of your target zone (50 percent). Gradually build up to the higher part of your target zone (75 percent). After six months of regular exercise, you may be able to exercise comfortably at up to 85 percent of your maximum heart rate.

D. Improve Heart Health

We know that regular exercise benefits the cardiovascular system. It strengthens your heart and improves circulation. It increases endurance and lowers blood pressure. It assists in losing unwanted weight. Working at a lower heart rate provides more fat-burning benefits while higher rates provide cardiovascular benefits. Walking, biking, jogging, and swimming are all beneficial exercises. It would be smart to do something every day. If you are an inactive person and have a heart condition, please seek medical advice before beginning any exercise regimen. There are supervised medical athletic centers that provide professional supervision and monitoring during any exercise program. Many of these places are geared toward people who are recovering from heart surgery or have medical conditions that may lead to heart problems.

In my view, machines at health clubs are not that accurate in measuring heart rate. You can purchase a heart rate monitor on the internet or through sporting goods or biking stores. It looks like a watch and can be worn anywhere (prices and models vary). A monitor can help you keep track of not only your heart rate, but also your target zone and calories burned.

For example: if you are fifty years old, your target maximum working heart rate would be 170 beats per minute. When you begin your workout regimen, aim for a consistent level of eighty-five and gradually work up to about 127. When you've maintained this level for six months or more, you may comfortably work up to 144.

E. Lower Cholesterol

There are two types of cholesterol: low density lipoprotein (LDL) ''bad'' cholesterol, which can damage the arteries and thus lead to heart disease, and high-density lipoprotein (HDL) which in higher amounts can transport the excess LDL into the liver where it is then transported out of the body. Cholesterol particle size varies. It appears that the larger protein particles are increased during exercise, reducing the harmful smaller particles. Therefore, when we exercise, we lower our "bad" cholesterol count. A study from Duke University Medical Center and East Carolina University tested 111 inactive, overweight men and women. People who exercised at least thirty minutes a day were able to lower their LDL rate. The ones who added more vigorous exercise which amounted to up to twenty miles a week of jogging not only lowered LDL but also increased HDL rates. It is possible to jog twenty miles a week on a treadmill, putting in just three miles per day for six to seven days.

F. Prevent Diabetes 2 (Adult-Onset Diabetes)

In this form of diabetes, the pancreas produces more insulin while sugar builds up in the bloodstream. Genetics, obesity, high LDL levels, smoking, inactive lifestyle, and diet play an integral role in whether a person may be diagnosed with diabetes 2. Moderate exercise can help burn excess weight and improve the use of insulin in the body. The body requires extra fuel (glucose) during moderate exercise, which will lower blood sugar. Aerobics, strength training, swimming, walking, and biking in moderate amounts have all shown to be of benefit for diabetics. However, if you have been diagnosed with diabetes, please consult with your doctor on which level of exercise is appropriate and on how you can monitor your insulin level, medicines, and diet. According to the Centers for Disease Control and Prevention's National Diabetes Fact Sheet, over 23 million people over the age of twenty were diagnosed with diabetes 2 in 2007. This disease became the seventh leading cause of death in North America in 2006.

G. Prevent Alzheimer's

Exercise has mental benefits, too. Recent research has shown that regular exercise may not only prevent diabetes and heart disease, but it may also help prevent dementia and Alzheimer's (AD). Walking, stationary biking, gardening, and swimming can help to boost mood, keep the body strong, and avoid other health problems. Since brain damage may start ten to twenty years before an AD diagnosis, preventive measures are so important. If a family member has been diagnosed with Alzheimer's, please consult with your doctor. The National Institute on Aging states that over 4.5 million Americans have AD, with that number doubling every five years because of the number of people living over the age of 65.

The Chinese Body Chart

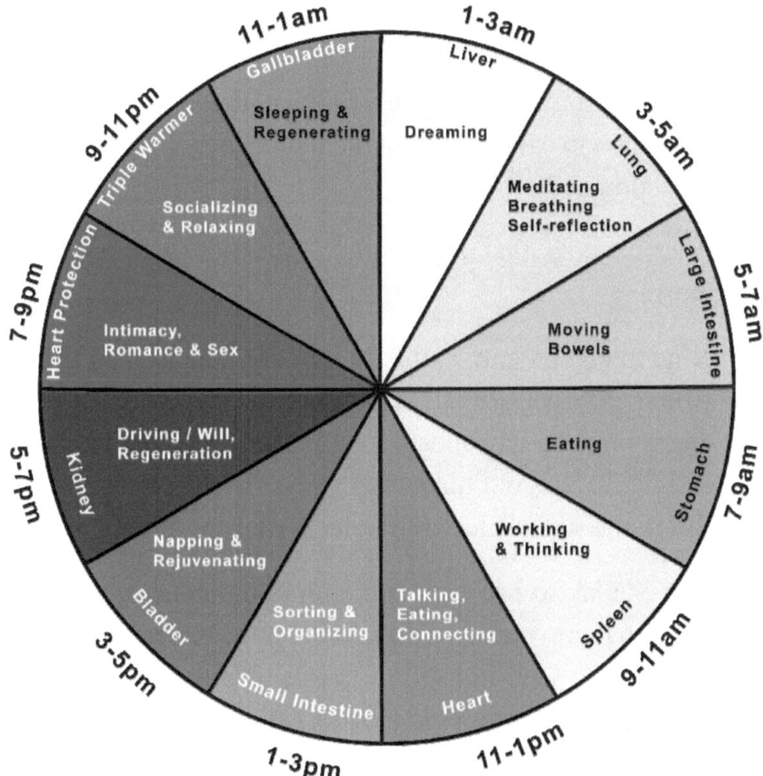

Chinese medicine has always been at the top of my list of things to do if I feel like I need some "good" medicine. This is a 5,000-year-old science for treating the body. The Chinese chart is fascinating, as well as so informative. The twenty-four-hour cycle is divided into twelve, two-hour intervals. The chart shows us different times to eat, rest, have sex, and sleep, as well as support our organs. The chart is made up of twelve meridians, which are minute pathways along which energy circulates. They are composed of yin and yang. The yin group consists of lungs, heart area, heart, kidney, liver, and spleen, whereas the yang group consists of the large intestine, small intestine, stomach, and bladder.

- Five a.m. to seven a.m. is the time of the large intestine, making it a perfect time to have a bowel movement and remove toxins from the day before. It is believed that combing your hair helps to clear out energy from the mind. At this time, emotions of defensiveness or feelings of being stuck could be evoked.

- Seven to nine a.m. is the time of the stomach, so it is important to eat the biggest meal of the day here to optimize digestion and absorption.
- Warm meals that are high in nutrition are best in the morning.
- Nine to eleven a.m. is the time of the pancreas and spleen, where enzymes are released to help digest food and release energy for the day ahead. This is the ideal time to exercise and work. Do your most taxing tasks of the day at this time. Emotions such as low self-esteem may be felt at this time.
- Eleven a.m. to one p.m. is the time of the heart, which will work to pump nutrients around the body to help provide you with energy and nutrition. This is also a good time to eat lunch and it is recommended to have a light, cooked meal. Having a one-hour nap or a cup of tea is also recommended during this time. Feelings of extreme joy or sadness can also be experienced at this time.
- One to three p.m. is the time of the small intestine and is when food eaten earlier will complete its digestion and assimilation. This is also a good time to go about daily tasks or exercise. Sometimes, vulnerable thoughts or feelings of abandonment may subconsciously arise at this time.
- Three to five p.m. is the time of the bladder, when metabolic wastes move into the kidney's filtration system. This is the perfect time to study or complete brain-challenging work. Another cup of tea is advised as is drinking a lot of water to help aid detoxification processes. Feeling irritated or timid

may also occur at this time.

- Five to seven p.m. is the time of the kidneys, when the blood is filtered, and the kidneys work to maintain proper chemical balance. This is the perfect time to have dinner and to activate your circulation, by walking, having a massage or stretching. Subconscious thoughts of fear or terror can also be active at this time.

- Seven to nine p.m. is the time of circulation, when nutrients are carried to the capillaries and to each cell. This is the perfect time to read. Avoid doing mental activities at this time. A difficulty in expressing emotions may also be felt; however, this is the perfect time to have sex or conceive.

- Nine to eleven p.m. is the time of the triple heater or endocrine system, where the body's homeostasis is adjusted, and enzymes are replenished. It is recommended to sleep at this time so the body can conserve energy for the following day. Feelings of paranoia or confusion may also be felt.

- Eleven p.m. to one a.m. is the time of the gallbladder and in order to wake feeling energized the body should be at rest. In Chinese medicine, this period of time is when yin energy fades, and yang energy begins to grow. Yang energy helps you to keep active during the day and is stored when you are asleep. Subconscious feelings of resentment may appear during this time.

- One to three a.m. is the time of the liver and a time when the body should be asleep. During this time, toxins are released from the body and fresh blood is made. If you find yourself waking during this time, you could have too much yang energy or problems with your liver or detoxification pathways. This is also the time of anger, frustration, and rage.

- Three to five a.m. is the time of the lungs and again, this is the time where the body should be asleep. If awake at this time, nerve-soothing exercises are recommended, such as breathing exercises. The body should be kept warm at this time too to help the lungs replenish the body with oxygen. The lungs are also associated with feelings of grief and sadness.

The above information comes from www.worldofhealth365.com.

There is a Chinese book that I bought in 1985. Dr. Stephen T. Chang is the author of *The Great Tao*. The book contains a multitude of golden wisdom, which I have read and re-read. Dr. Chang writes about the Tao of philosophy and revitalization of internal exercises. He discusses nutrition and the balanced diet. The book also includes health conditions, sexual wisdom, and the I-Ching. There are exercises shown which coordinate with the twelve meridians. Each two-hour period is displayed with an exercise to support, balance, and energize the specific organs. We have all experienced a disruption in our biorhythm (biological clock). Our biorhythm regulates our energy in relationship to our solar and lunar time. One example of disruptive energy is when we travel through different time zones (jet fatigue). Being aware of the Chinese clock and Dr. Chang's specific exercises adds more support and vitality for our bodies.

There's clearly an inverse relationship between the amount of exercise and the number of (plaque) deposits in the brain. Exercise changes the body's reaction to forming deposits; additional blood flow to the brain may help flush away the plaque.

—Sangram Sisodia
Professor of Neurosciences, University of Chicago

Start Moving!

If you had more vitality, better health, a more positive outlook, and an improved immune system, would you feel differently about yourself? If your depression lifted, heart disease, cancer, diabetes, and obesity didn't exist, and your energy level was higher than you could have ever imagined, how would you feel? If aches and pains disappeared and your body became stronger and more flexible, wouldn't it give you a new lease on life? It's never too late to rejuvenate ourselves; we can start now.

As mentioned above by Professor Sangram Sisodia, recent research has shown that regular exercise may not only prevent diabetes and heart disease, but actually may help prevent dementia and Alzheimer's.

Those benefits alone make it all worthwhile. But before you join your local fitness center and dive into a new exercise program, check with your health practitioner, especially if you haven't been physically active in a while.

Get Moving!

As we age, our metabolism slows. To remain fit, we need to balance daily exercise, a healthy diet (preferably full of alkaline foods), proper rest, and joyful intentions. Bob Greene, Oprah Winfrey's trainer promotes overall fitness and says that functional fitness is a person's ability to first perform exercises and movements effectively; cardio, and muscle training comprise the other two-thirds of an overall fitness program.

Core training, strengthening, aerobics, and flexibility are my key areas of focus. I rarely get injured or sore, I sleep better, and my weight stays where I want it. Depression lifts and life is exhilarating. Feeling sexy and desirable in the later years is an added bonus. Why not?

Getting Started

1. Be Patient

When you make a commitment to exercising, you will find the first two weeks are the biggest hurdle. Muscle soreness or just plain weariness may discourage you from sticking with your program. If you manage to exercise for just one month, you have a much better chance of staying with it for life. When you have reached the one-month benchmark, re-evaluate your regimen, and see how you can perform in different and more challenging ways.

2. Start with Something You Enjoy

It could be as simple as a fifteen-minute walk three times a week, building up to a thirty-minute walk, five days a week. Don't try to start at the top; building up to thirty minutes of exercise a day is safer and encourages you to stay consistent. Years ago, Jane Fonda, along with other fitness instructors, advocated continuing the workout to the point of exhausting the muscles, thus creating the feeling of muscles "burning." That "burn theory" is now passé. You will not receive any more benefits working out for an hour than you will for thirty minutes.

3. Join a Club/Find a Partner

I encourage you to join a club in your neighborhood rather than investing in expensive equipment for your home that will likely wind up decorating your garage or basement. Also, working out with other people can be stimulating. The "buddy system" should encourage both of you to show up and help you keep to your regimen.

One of the most challenging parts of exercise is sticking with a program and feeling good about reaching certain goals—be it weight loss, strength and flexibility, exercising your heart and circulatory system, or simply getting in shape.

4. Consider a Personal Trainer

A good fitness club (including your local YMCA) employs professional trainers who will help you develop a fitness regimen tailored to your needs. So, make a plan; work with a trainer three to five times when you begin. If you suffer from arthritis or other joint problems, begin your fitness program with a qualified person trained in physical therapy who has a good overall knowledge of arthritis and other joint problems.

If a personal trainer is not the way you wish to initially start, familiarize yourself with the equipment, ask questions, and by all means, join others in core training, yoga, or Pilates classes. You will learn more about your body, have fun with others, and be inspired to continue your quest to becoming a healthier person.

5. Mix It Up

Variety is the spice of life. I see the same people doing the same exercises over and over and they look bored to tears while they talk on their cell phones. My suggestion is to try different things and decide which ones you delight in. I enjoy cross-training, which I call "mixing it up." One day I may decide to go for a swim on the day I normally take a fitness class. I don't get bored, and my body says, "Oh, this is something new." It's super beneficial and so enjoyable.

6. Ways to Exercise

There are multitudes of ways to exercise. In the age of super technology, the latest invention is the Wii™ video game with workouts and balance choices. For instance, I watched a granddaughter play singles tennis with her younger sister using a control to hit the ball back and forth on the court.

In my day, I needed an actual racket, court, outfit, and partner to play the game.

I purchase yoga and Pilates DVDs on the internet. They come in handy when I wish to fit in a workout without going out my front door. This section will give you a taste of different forms of exercise and their benefits. I'll cover workout equipment, Pilates, walking, yoga, water aerobics, dance, and tai chi.

What to Eat When Exercising

Exercising on an empty stomach can cause glucose stores to become low and create low blood sugar (hypoglycemia), which may result in dizziness or headaches. You risk breaking down muscle protein to provide needed carbohydrates to your body during exercise. Before your workout, eat bread, cereal, and fruit. They provide the energy needed for an hour workout. If your workout is longer, within an hour following a workout, make a whey protein drink which contains 20 grams (g) of whey protein. It is most important to consume whey protein immediately after your exercise session to make sure adequate protein is available to depleted muscles. Another protein suggestion is a turkey, tomato, lettuce sandwich to help rebuild muscle tissue and stimulate the immune system. Don't forget to re-hydrate with water.

A. Aerobic and Anaerobic Demystified

Aerobic exercise, such as running, provides more oxygen to your muscles and burns more calories than weightlifting. Aerobic exercise includes endurance activities such as marathon running or distance biking, walking, swimming, and cross-country skiing. Aerobic exercise also reduces chances of hip fractures, improves circulation, increases lung capacity, and lowers blood pressure. It helps to increase the size of the heart muscle while providing a lower resting heart rate, thereby benefiting the entire cardiovascular system and reducing cardiovascular disease. Aerobic exercising for twenty to thirty minutes three to four times a week reduces body fat and the risk of diabetes. It also increases HDL (good) cholesterol, decreases LDL (bad) cholesterol, and promotes a longer, healthier life.

Remember to aim at the lowest part of your target zone and gradually build up to the higher part of your target zone.

Anaerobic exercise includes weight training, tennis, and sprinting. Anything that requires short bursts of high intensity exertion is considered anaerobic. Weight training, an anaerobic exercise, helps make stronger bones, increases muscle strength and mass, and reduces age-related muscle atrophy. It also contributes to weight loss, though not as much as aerobic exercise. Falls occur more frequently for those over 65, so doesn't it make sense to strengthen your muscles?

Workout Drinks

Sports drinks are only necessary during a workout if you are exercising for ninety minutes or longer. They maximize fluid absorption and enhance performance by delivering carbohydrates and electrolytes, the most crucial of which is sodium. Sports drinks designed for use during exercise typically contain a combination of simple carbohydrates (sucrose, glucose, and fructose) and complex carbohydrates, such as glucose polymers and maltodextrins. The better-formulated drinks usually contain both, with a higher percentage of complex carbohydrates rather than simple carbohydrates.

Massage

I have had massages for many years and have friends who are certified therapists. My body has experienced hot stones, Rolfing, shiatsu, Swedish, Hawaiian lomilomi, reflexology, cranial sacral and Thai massages. When I lived near hot springs, I would soak to loosen up tight muscles and then head for my bodywork, which lasted sixty to ninety minutes. I try to schedule massages twice a month, especially when I am working hard on a book project or after a strenuous hike.

Let's Talk Massage Therapy

My dear friend, Chandler McLay, became a certified massage therapist in 1996. Her other talents include guiding women's spiritual wilderness trips and working with young people and their families regarding addiction therapy. Chandler shared with me the modalities and benefits of massage therapy:

> "Massage is one of the oldest remedial techniques in dealing with healing. It is also perhaps the most natural and instinctive means to relieve pain. There are accounts of massage as a healing art going back to the Chinese Amma Techniques of 3,000 BC. Massage is mentioned in Japanese, Indian, Greek, Roman, and Arabic histories. A review of the writings of Hippocrates indicates he believed all physicians should be trained in massage. Yet, as modern western medicine became popular, many of these historic references to simple healing arts drifted into the background. Fortunately, they are now experiencing a long-overdue recognition of their physical, emotional, and spiritual value.
>
> "It is the responsibility of each individual to become active in his/her own healing, regardless of the modality. If you choose massage as one of your healing options, I recommend you find a reputable spa or an individual therapist recommended by a reliable friend, or go to a clinic offered by a massage school. Enjoy a one-hour full-body massage. Massage may be light or very deep. What does your body need? Want? Have you experienced any injuries recently or had surgery? Are you feeling depressed, sore, too heavy, or embarrassed about the shape your body is in? All these considerations will affect the quality of your relationship to your own healing. When you find a massage therapist you feel comfortable with, you will be able to simply get more deeply in touch with yourself. Professional body work often releases old traumas and dramas; that is part of its value and healing quality. Thus, I emphasize the importance of finding a therapist with whom you feel confident and comfortable."

Once you have experienced two or three general massages, you may want to be adventurous and try other varieties of body work. Read about them, ask your massage therapist about them, ask your natural health-care adviser about them, and find what feels good for you.

Paybacks for Massage

- Improved circulation
- Lymph movement
- Detoxification
- Release of lactic acid after strenuous activity
- Possible improvement of blood pressure
- Pain relief
- Relaxation
- Improved flexibility
- Lubrication and exfoliation of the skin
- Emotional release
- Spiritual connection

B. Weight Training—Making Muscle Work for You

Muscle is metabolically active, meaning it requires a lot of calories to do its thing; we burn calories by increasing our metabolism. One hour of lifting weights can burn up to 450 calories. People who want to lose weight focus on aerobic activity, although weight training can help offset our slowing metabolism and is as productive in creating a leaner body as cardiovascular activity. While cardio training may burn more calories, weight training provides stronger muscles to help ward off osteoporosis.

I completed a six-week session of weight training at my health club while writing this book. The trainer worked with me for an hour each session. Even though I had been lifting weights and using the machines, he introduced me to an entirely new way of strengthening and shaping. I now feel more confident that I can achieve maximum benefit in a thirty- to forty-five-minute workout by following his guidelines. I plan to work out with this new program for a couple of months and then may go back for another session with the trainer to see what else I can achieve.

As we grow older, it is impossible for women to develop bulk as men do; however, weight training helps men and women tone and shape muscles, maintain flexibility, and prevent osteoporosis.

Paybacks

- Burn calories.
- Strengthen bones.
- Improve flexibility.
- Prevent osteoporosis.

Workout Guidelines

- Warm up by s t r e t c h i n g your body.
- Don't consume food while exercising.
- Drink plenty of water.
- Sign up for a training session before using the equipment and use it wisely.
- Use stretching to cool down after workout.

C. Walk On

This is one simple exercise you can do anywhere. During the winter months, I use the treadmill and on beautiful, sunshiny days I head outside for an hour walk. According to a groundbreaking study at the Erasmus MC University Medical Center in Rotterdam, walking at a moderate pace for thirty minutes a day, five days a week delays cardiovascular disease and increases your lifespan nearly four years. Walking helps boost the metabolism and helps prevents colorectal cancer in men. You can walk on treadmills, bike and jogging paths, around your neighborhood, or wherever you desire. Adding light hand weights and walking at a brisk pace stimulates the metabolism, makes your muscles leaner and keeps the weight off. The cardiovascular benefits for the heart and blood are superb. There are so many benefits from so little time and energy spent. And it's so simple and fun. To lose weight and keep it off, you need to get moving. You will raise your HDL (good cholesterol) and get the blood pumping through your circulatory system. You can walk with a group or by yourself. Don't forget to bring your water bottle to stay hydrated.

Paybacks

- Helps burn fat.
- Cancer preventive for healthier heart, colon, and breasts.
- Makes muscles leaner.
- Increases blood through circulatory system.

D. Elliptical Trainers—Anaerobic

I use this machine for at least thirty minutes or cross-train ten minutes on the elliptical, stationary bike, and treadmill—providing a complete thirty-minute cardio workout. For those who have not used them before, elliptical trainers or "cross trainers" look like a cross between a treadmill and a step machine. As your feet move on the pedals, your legs go through an elliptical movement, reducing pounding and stress on joints in the legs, hips, and back. This machine works very well to stimulate the cardiovascular system. It strengthens the quads, hamstrings, and gluteus and, if using the upper body attachments, the biceps, triceps, chest, and back.

Paybacks

- Strengthens leg muscles.
- Strengthens arms, back, and chest.
- Raises heart rate to burn fat.
- Increases oxygen level.

E. Stair Stepper—Aerobic

Stair steppers, or climbers, are excellent machines to burn calories and exercise the major muscle groups of the lower body. Look for sturdy, padded handrails to help balance, electronic programs to keep you interested, and easy-to-set resistance settings. A sturdy steel or aluminum frame is a must. The best stair climbers keep your feet on an even plane with the floor at all times, allowing natural foot articulation. While there is a fundamental simplicity in the stair climbing exercise itself, add-on accessories for the upper body can provide a total body workout. Plus, stepping or climbing can be a rigorous exercise just by the sheer effort it takes. An all-out workout on a stair climber can consume as much energy as you are capable of producing. Besides using it regularly, try to get the maximum benefit from the machine by taking big steps and using the handrails only for light support. For a more difficult workout, let go of the rails every now and then—but take care not to lose your balance. Users who do not grip the handrails will burn upward of 20 percent more calories per workout than those who lean heavily on the rails.

Paybacks

- Burns calories.
- Strengthens leg muscles.
- Increases healthy heart benefits.
- Promotes more oxygen to lungs.

F. Treadmill

Many people like the low impact of treadmills (easier on the knees), and the fact that they let you walk about as fast as you want to, or even run. While running has been a favored activity of Americans since the 1970s, walking has come into vogue in the last several years, in part because it's an exercise that older or less-fit people can do easily.

Whether you walk or run on a treadmill, it's an activity with numerous physical benefits. Many people have gotten used to using the treadmills in their health clubs and YMCAs. Of course, treadmill technology is constantly changing and improving. In the past few years, a few manufacturers have come out with treadmills featuring electric inclines that adjust automatically, based on feedback from the unit's heart rate monitor.

Paybacks

- Great for the cardiovascular system.
- Improves the heart, lungs, and circulatory system.
- An efficient way to lose body fat.
- Since it's a weight-bearing activity, it has musculoskeletal benefits as well.

G. Recumbent Bike

If plagued by lower back pain, consider recumbent bikes. They have cushioned chair-like seats and pedals in front which offer better support for the lower back than regular bikes. The downside is you may find yourself going more slowly and easily than you would on an upright model, which means the workout won't be as difficult. You'll need to really push yourself to stay in your target heart rate zone. I vary between the recumbent bikes and the upright stationary bikes. During beautiful weather, I bike outside.

Biking Down the Open Road

Everywhere you go, people are biking. It may be a ride to do errands or just a pleasant day to spend outside feeling the cool breeze on your face. There are serious bikers who do single track in the mountains too. When I was young, I rode my bike to school practically every day. I still ride as part of staying physically fit. I have a bike that has several gears for going up and down the hills, as well as a women's bike seat that is comfortable for longer rides. It is important to have a water carrier so that you keep hydrated, especially on warm days. Have a bike helmet that fits you well and biking gloves to keep your hands from slipping. Bicycling is an aerobic exercise, which means that your heart, blood vessels, and lungs all get a workout. Studies show that regular cycling cuts risk of heart disease by 50 percent. Cycling also is easier on the joints than pounding the hard ground. It has a fifth of the impact on your body that jogging does. Cycling several days of week for thirty minutes or more will provide a multitude of health benefits.

Paybacks

- Tones legs.
- Burns calories.
- Look younger with healthier skin.
- Easier on joints than running.
- Increases strength and stamina.
- Increases energy levels.
- Adds more brain cells.
- Strengthens bones.
- Decreases body fat levels.
- Reduces anxiety and depression.
- Strengthens heart.

- Assists people with handicaps or missing limbs.
- Helps people with joint, back, or balance challenges.

Types of Bikes

- Catrike recumbent—more comfortable for people who are older and who have had neck, wrist, and hand strains while riding a regular bike.
- Electric pedal-assist bikes—kicks in when you need a break from pedaling.

Paybacks

- Strengthens legs.
- Cardio benefits by increasing the tension.
- Burns calories.
- Using light hand weights increases upper body strength.

H. Yoga from the Heart

Yoga, or the Sanskrit translation "union," is an ancient practice—believed to be at least five thousand years old. During my early thirties, I was raising five young children and couldn't afford the luxury of taking formal classes, let alone find a sitter to take care of the brood. I self-practiced yoga for years before stopping in favor of distance running. When I was in my forties my back seized up and I found myself crawling to a yoga class in California. My teacher taught the Iyengar method of yoga, which is initially learned through the in-depth study of asanas (postures) and pranayama (breath control). We used props to help open various parts of the body. I found the class extremely intense but was determined to go twice a week. At times, my lower back would ache so much I told the instructor I didn't want to continue. She assured me that if I made a commitment to stay with it, I would experience relief and improvement—which I did after four to six months. To this day, in my eighties, the pain has not returned.

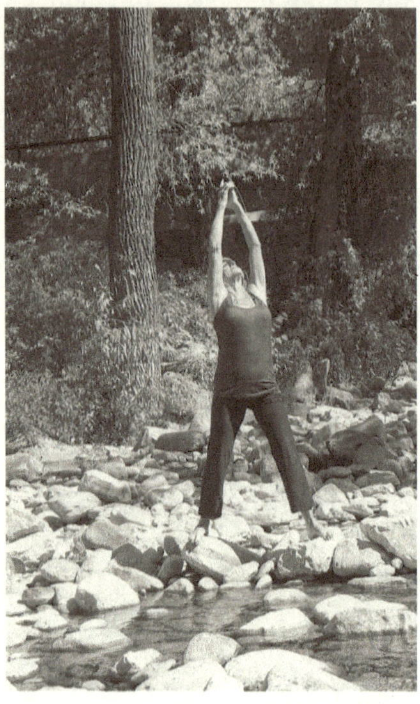

Another teacher, Hollis, recently told me that "By practicing yoga, you learn to connect with your body and listen to all of its wonderful messages. More importantly, you begin to accept the changes in your body and respect your limitations. This will be a huge lesson." My teacher's words resonate loud and clear, and I have more understanding of my injuries and the physical activities I include in my daily life. While taking a yoga class with my daughter, who is in her forties, a teacher mentioned that I was the "elder" in the room. The instructor told the vibrant men and women in their thirties that we can stay flexible our entire lives. I may be in my seventies, but my inner voice keeps reminding me that I still feel youthful.

Paybacks

- Standing postures strengthen and lengthen muscles, making them less prone to injury.

- Weight-bearing postures help the body deposit more calcium into bones and joints.
- Inverted postures direct blood and other vital fluids to specific body parts, glands, and organs and regulate hormones.
- Certain postures aid in digestion and elimination.
- Spine twisting postures cause the discs between the vertebrae to act as sponges soaking in blood and fluids.
- Yoga's breathing techniques increase lung capacity and help quiet and focus the mind.

Kundalini Yoga

I find this form of yoga exhilarating, and practice at home for thirty to sixty minutes depending on my day. It blends well with traditional yoga classes. The breath work and simple movements are transformational.

Paybacks

- Teaches breathing through the nose.
- Works the abdominal area.
- Sends healing energy up through the spine.
- Improves the function of the liver, adrenals, heart, kidneys, and lungs.
- Gives an inner peace and outer strength.
- Creates boundless energy.

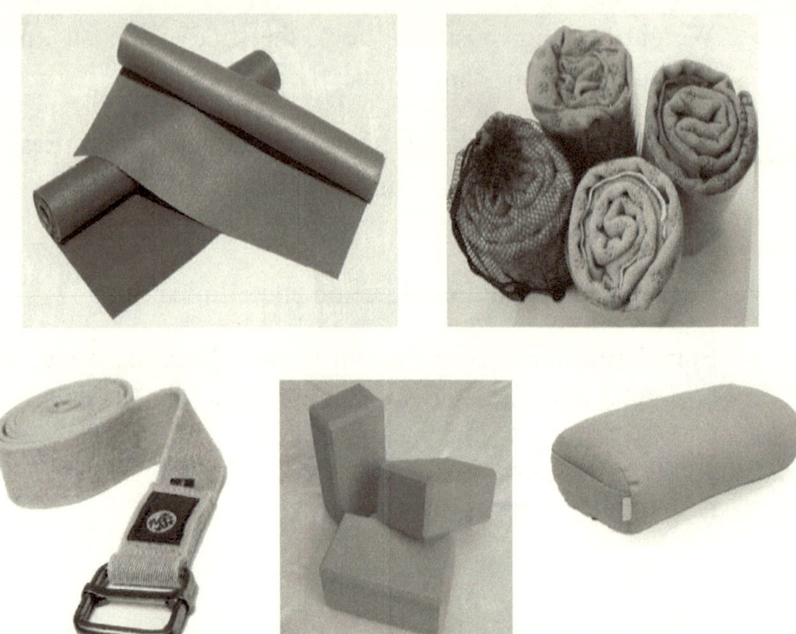

Examples of Yoga Props: Mats, Blankets, Belt, Blocks, and Bolster

I. Pilates

I must be right. Never an aspirin. Never injured a day in my life. The whole country, the whole world, should be doing my exercises. They'd be happier.

—Joseph Hubertus Pilates, in 1965, age 86.

I took my first Pilates mat class when I was fifty-nine. I had heard about Pilates, but frankly didn't know what to expect. I liked it, however, and continued on with other teachers, taking a variety of classes: mat, ballet routines, and the reformer machine. I have been athletic my entire life and relied on my muscles and not my core strength. Pilates was a major wake-up call for strengthening my postural muscles, which include muscles that wrap around your torso. It has made me more aware of my body and how it moves. I truly love doing Pilates. I take mat classes twice a week and use resistance tools such as the magic circle and resistance bands. Recently I have started reformer classes again, which consist of pulleys and springs that activate muscles differently than on the mat. When I lived in Hawaii my instructor was struck by a car while on her motorcycle, fracturing her fibula in two places and her tibia in two. Thanks to Pilates, she had an almost full recovery and was teaching one week after she left the hospital. She told me that Pilates has led her to an amazing way of movement and philosophy of being. The German man Joseph Pilates, the founder of Pilates, was a sickly child, which gave him the ambition to become healthy and strong. He became a skier, gymnast, boxer, and took up yoga. He taught his exercise methods to soldiers in hospitals during World War I. In 1926, Joseph Pilates came to the United States and began teaching ballet dancers, using mats and machines.

As with all new exercises, if you have chronic pain, please consult with your health-care practitioner before you attend a Pilates class. There are many books, tapes, and videos on the subject, but none of them can take the place of an instructor. Pilates is different in each person's body; an instructor can tell you where and how you should feel each movement. A private, one-on-one lesson with an instructor is the ideal; however, this is not an option for many—cost being one factor and finding a qualified instructor another.

Paybacks

- More flexibility
- More strength
- Increased range of motion
- More abdominal strength
- Better body awareness and coordination
- Total body workout
- Better posture

- More mobility
- Helps recovery from injuries

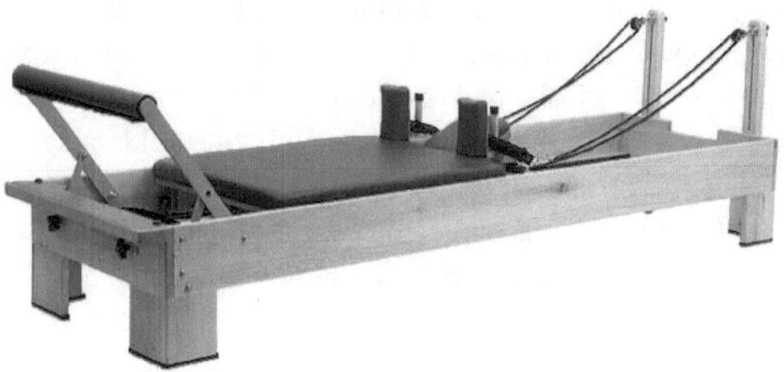

Pilates Reformer Machine

J. Water Aerobics

We're surrounded by life-giving fluid for nine months before our births, so doesn't it make sense to connect with water during our lifetime? I have been swimming since the age of three. While living in Hawaii, I swam in the beautiful Pacific Ocean. I got to witness dolphins, turtles, and reef fish swimming around me. I enjoyed the therapeutic benefits of salt water as well as hot springs. Our bodies contain 70 percent water, so when we are immersed in water, we relax our minds and bodies and feel better. A water aerobics instructor in Hawaii shared the following with me: "People of all ages and fitness can enjoy aqua classes. The water makes the body more buoyant, so we experience less stress on the joints. Therefore, those suffering from medical conditions such as neck or back pain, obesity, or joint aches can do the classes as well as more healthy individuals." When we are immersed in water, we reduce the pounding on bones, joints, and muscles; thus we experience less soreness and pain after a class. An ideal water temperature is eighty-three degrees Fahrenheit.

If you are uncomfortable about using weight training equipment, aqua aerobics is an excellent alternative. Water aerobics can be done in waist-to-chest-deep water or deeper if using a flotation jacket. There are a variety of movements and programs from beginning levels to advanced. If you are new to water aerobics, let your instructor know. Schedule a time to meet with your instructor to write up a plan, whether your goal is long-term or short.

Paybacks

- Improves strength and flexibility.
- Improves abdominal and back strength.
- Burns an average of 450-700 calories in one hour.
- Increases range of motion in knees and hips.
- You can train at your own pace, eliminating the need to compete.
- Safe environment for those who are not strong swimmers.
- Reduces pounding of joints, bones, and muscles.
- Cooler environment than on land.

What to Take to the Pool

- Aqua shoes are good for traction on the pool bottom and provide more stability.
- Buoys or aqua blocks (small barbells made for the water) increase resistance as you move your arms through the water.
- Flotation belts help free the lower body/legs for undisturbed motion and help with proper body alignment while in the water.
- Webbed gloves increase resistance.
- Kickboards are useful for lower body resistance.

Safety Measures

Check with your physician before planning any exercise regime. Some health insurance companies may cover the cost of an aqua class if prescribed by a doctor. Be sure to let the instructor know if this is your first aqua class.

If we seek the real source of the dance, if we go to nature, we find that the dance of the future is the dance of the past, the dance of eternity, and has been and always will be the same... The movement of waves, of winds, of the earth is ever the same lasting harmony.

—Isadora Duncan

K. Dance

I learned ballet as a child, rock and roll as a teenager, and progressed to jazz, NIA®, and Zumba® dancing as an adult.

Dance has become the rage among people of all ages, but especially baby boomers and older. Ballroom, hip-hop, swing, samba, tango, jazz, country & western, and even ballet classes are available in practically every town. Remember when dancing all night was fun and exhilarating? Dance provides so many benefits for both our physical bodies and our psyches. When we dance, we are able to lose ourselves in the rhythm and sensuous movement, leaving our troubles behind.

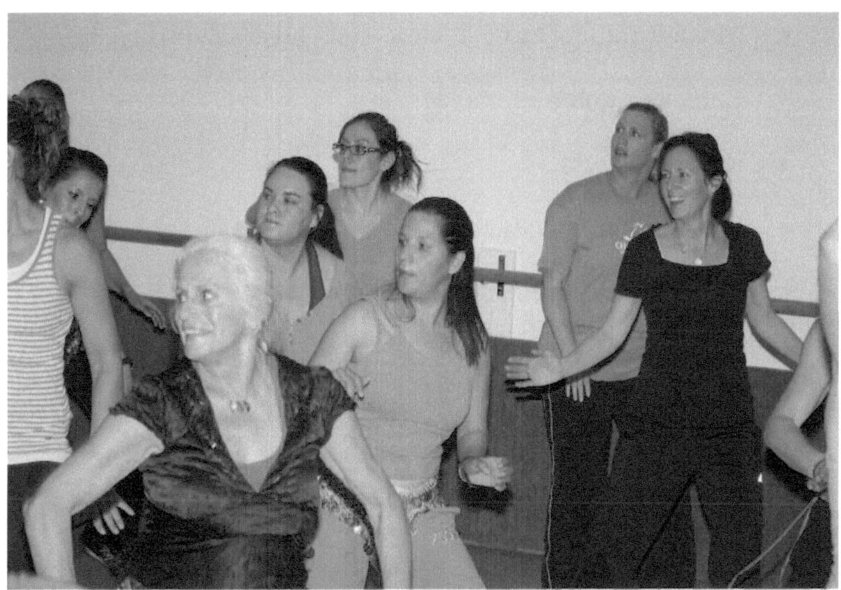

Zumba® is an exhilarating program. You get to boogie with easy movements to energizing music, often with Latin tempos. In the spring of 2010, the Zumba® program had 60,000 studios in 105 countries. Now, there are over 7.5 million participants taking Zumba classes every week.

The NIA Technique©, developed by Debbie and Carlos Rosa, provides aerobic and cardiovascular benefits, is a weight-bearing exercise, adds flexibility, and lubricates joints. Unlike many other exercise routines, dance requires no special equipment, and anyone can do it. The NIA Technique, because it is not choreographed, allows free expression in the movements. All levels are welcome.

Paybacks

- Enhances your social life.
- Raises self-confidence.
- Helps you meet new people and make new friends.
- Improves your overall heart, cardiovascular, and lung capacity.

- Makes you feel more at ease in social situations.
- Enhances grace and poise.
- Relieves stress.
- Slows aging process.
- Strengthens bones and helps prevent arthritis and osteoporosis.
- Burns calories.
- Is just plain fun.

L. Tai Chi

A few years ago, I was attending the American Booksellers Association conference in Chicago, Illinois. My hotel window overlooked Lake Michigan. One morning while preparing to go to the show, I watched a group of seniors practicing tai chi in a park near the lake. Their movements seemed effortless and beautiful to watch. I have taken tai chi lessons in nature-like settings, which I find more inspirational than inside classes.

Tai chi (tie-chee), an ancient martial art, can be performed by anyone. The slow, dance-like movement, accompanied by deep breathing, looks deceptively simple but can be a demanding, though most rewarding, discipline.

One out of every three seniors will experience a fall over the course of a year. In an Emory University study, people who participated in a tai chi class once a week and practiced twice a day cut their risks of falling by 50 percent. Our physical strength is greatly diminished by age fifty, and by age seventy we experience a one-third loss of strength in our lower extremities.

Paybacks

- Improves balance, lowers blood pressure, and reduces

stress.

- Helps with range of motion.
- Lubricates tendons and ligaments of the lower extremities, ankles, knees, and hips.
- Improves balance and coordination, bone strength, and elasticity.

M. Qigong (Ch'i Kung)

Qigong originates from Chinese martial arts and translates as "vital energy or life force." Before becoming well-known in western society, Qigong had been practiced in Buddhist and Taoist monasteries for health and spiritual benefits. In 2001 the Chinese government organized and formed the Chinese Health Qigong Association in affiliation with the Peking Sports University. Many regional colleges offer classes in Qigong as part of their school curriculum. I learned some of the movements simply because it incorporates breathing and movement techniques which flow easily, and I do notice an increase in chi energy throughout my body. Persons of any age can perform these movements which contain great health and body-mind-spirit connections.

Paybacks

- Reduces stress.
- Builds stamina and increases vitality.
- Enhances the immune system.
- Improves cardiovascular, respiratory, circulatory, lymphatic, and digestive functions.

N. Rebounder/Trampoline

A trampoline/rebounder provides excellent exercise and is just great fun. It stimulates all of your seventy-five trillion cells while strengthening your body at the same time. I have a small sturdy rebounder purchased at K-Mart for $15. I jump on it just ten minutes a day, usually while listening to music. If you have difficulty with balance, there are rebounders with a bar you can hold onto. If you don't have a place for a small trampoline, bouncing for ten minutes while sitting on the side of your bed is also beneficial.

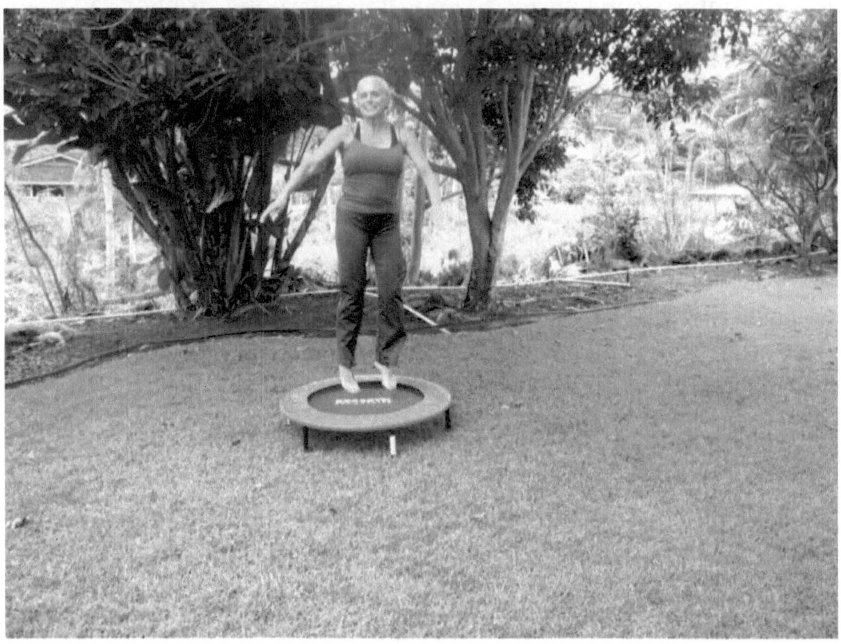

Paybacks

- Circulates oxygen to your tissues.
- Stimulates metabolism.
- Firms muscles, reducing obesity.
- Provides more energy & lessens fatigue.
- Improves vision.
- Aids in lymphatic circulation.
- Lowers cholesterol and triglycerides.

- Improves digestion and elimination.
- Strengthens heart and body muscles.
- Increases balance and coordination.
- Increases red blood cell count.
- Reduces headaches and other pain.
- Improves immune system.
- Slows aging process.

O. Inversion Table

An inversion table, sometimes referred to as spinal traction, has great benefits for many people. To use this device, one straps the feet in then lies back until the head drops toward. Users report that it helps decompress the vertebrae that get packed down over time. The same benefits are reported with special boots that hook over a bar.

As we age, gravity weighs us down, resulting in poor posture, weak stomach muscles (our core), and back pain. Our spine compresses, so we also become shorter by as much as two inches. It is not uncommon to see older people hunched over as if preparing to go back into the womb. Years ago, while visiting the Cayman Islands, our group took a boat trip to an outer island to visit an artist's studio. Although I was only in my early thirties at the time, one of the sculptures left an indelible impression: it was a man aging through the cycles of life, starting out as a fresh newborn, then an adult standing straight and tall, and finally ending as a crouched-over old man.

More Paybacks

- Studies have shown that within ten seconds, back pain decreases by 35 percent; the spine assumes its proper "S" curve and posture improves.

- Helps stimulate circulation.
- Helps balance awareness and motion sickness by stimulating the inner ear.
- Maintains internal organs in normal position, avoiding “prolapse” (to fall out of place).
- Increases oxygen to the brain.
- Helps reverse the effects of gravity.
- Relieves back pain.
- Reduces stress.
- Strengthens and elongates the spine.
- Allows more space between the vertebrae and relieves pressure on discs.
- Helps relax tense muscles.
- Speeds the flow of lymphatic fluids which flush out the body’s wastes and carry them to the bloodstream.
- Introduces fresh supplies of oxygen.
- Helps stiffness and muscle pain disappear.

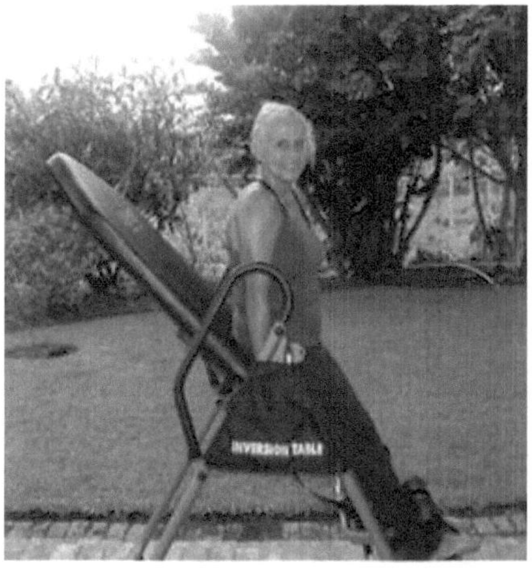

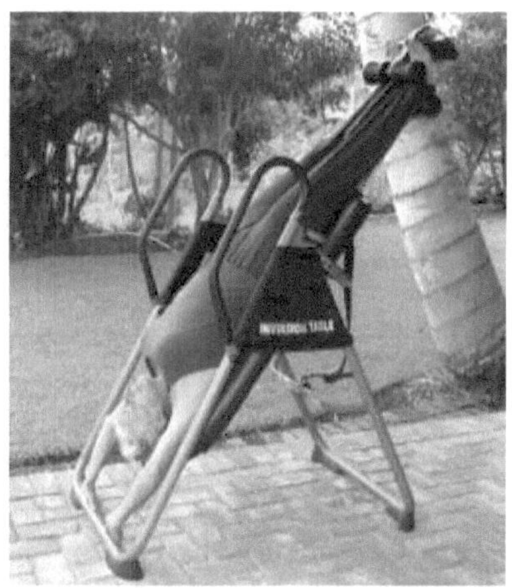

There are smaller inversion chairs available, and you may be able to obtain one with a physician's script and your health insurance. Always consult with a physician before you use an inversion table, especially if you have high blood pressure or other conditions.

P. The Tibetan Five Rites

These exercises were introduced into the West by a retired British Army colonel who discovered the much fabled and sought after Fountain of Youth at a remote monastery in the Himalayas. The rites enhance the flow of the subtle but powerful life force that circulates throughout the reproductive, adrenal, thymus, thyroid, pineal, and pituitary glands. Each rite is done as many times as comfortable at first and then the number of repetitions is gradually built up to twenty-one per day. While doing the exercises, it is extremely beneficial to breathe in deeply through the nose and exhale with vigor through the mouth during each repetition.

The First Rite

Stand and spin clockwise. Your arms are extended straight out to the sides. This enhances the flow of life force through the body. Initially, you may feel dizzy. One way to keep from getting dizzy is to hold your arms out from your body and focus attention on the thumbs.

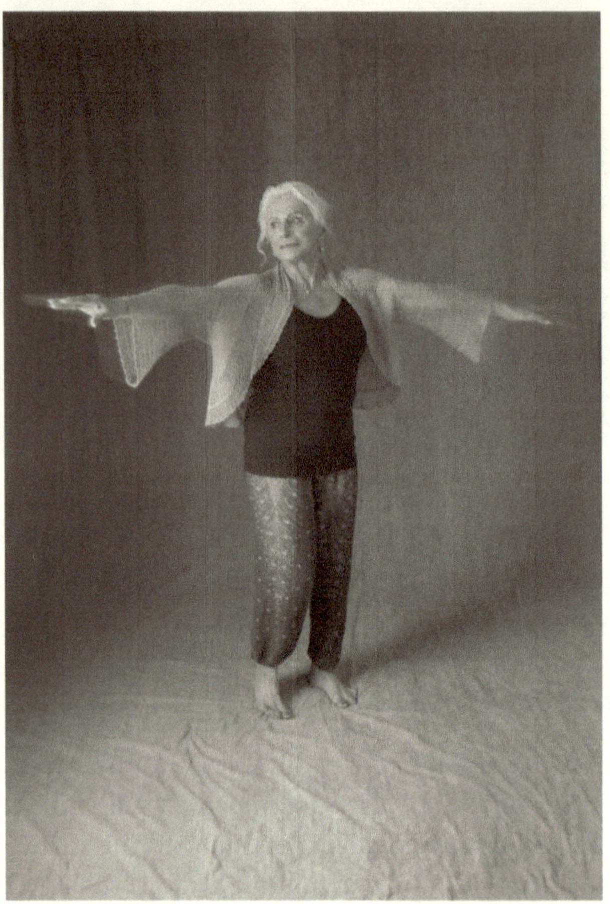

The Second Rite

Lie on your back with your arms to your sides. The head lifts to the chest while the legs stretch straight up into the air. Then lower the head and legs. At first this movement may seem difficult for keeping the legs straight; however, with time you will improve and find it much easier. It is important to use the breath with all of these exercises. Concentrate on the abdominal region rather than the chest. Breathe in deeply through the nose as you raise the legs and exhale through the mouth as you lower the legs.

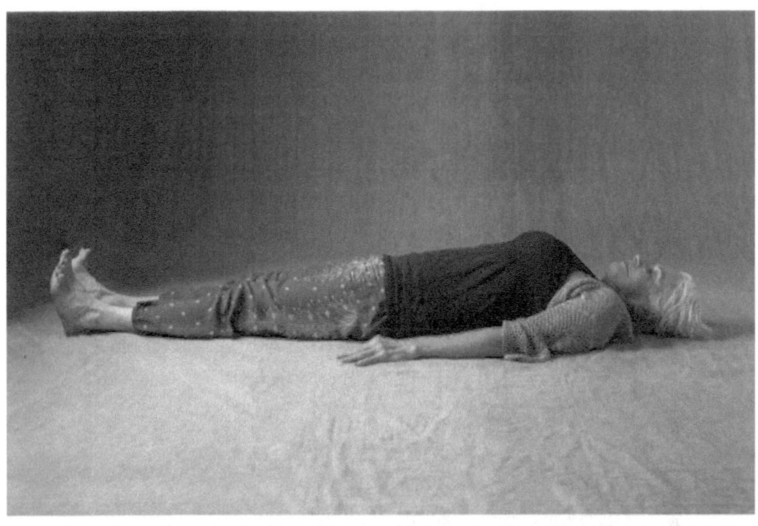

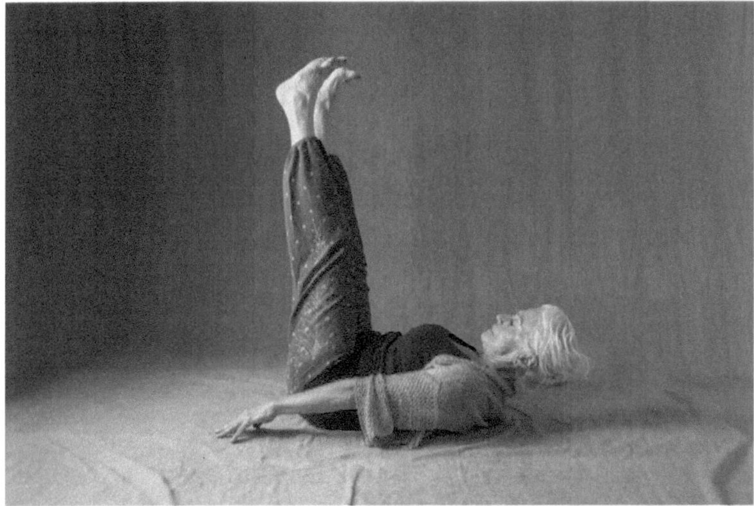

The Third Rite

Kneel on the floor with your arms by your side and your hands placed against your hamstrings.

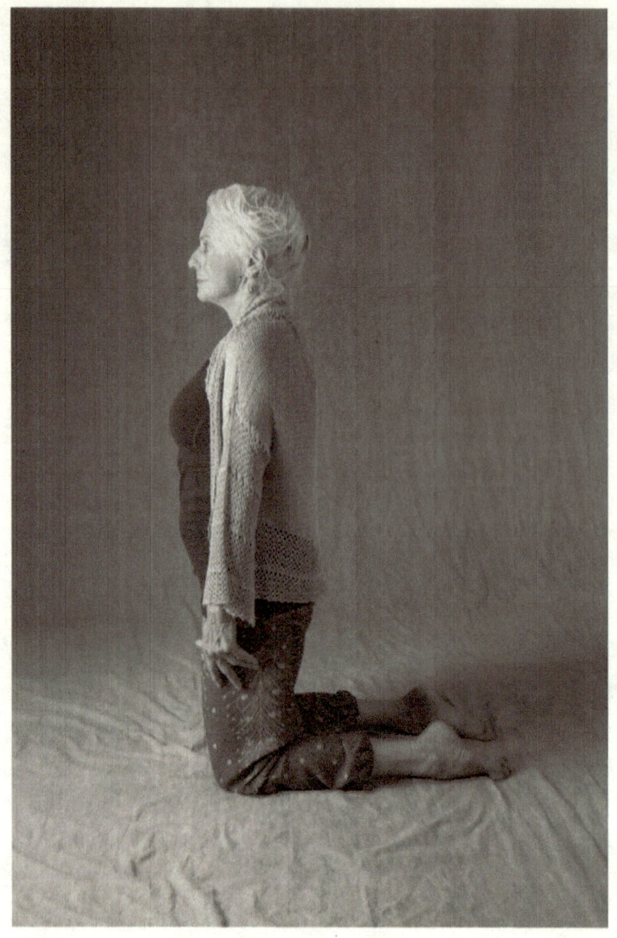

Bend the head forward while tucking the chin against your head.

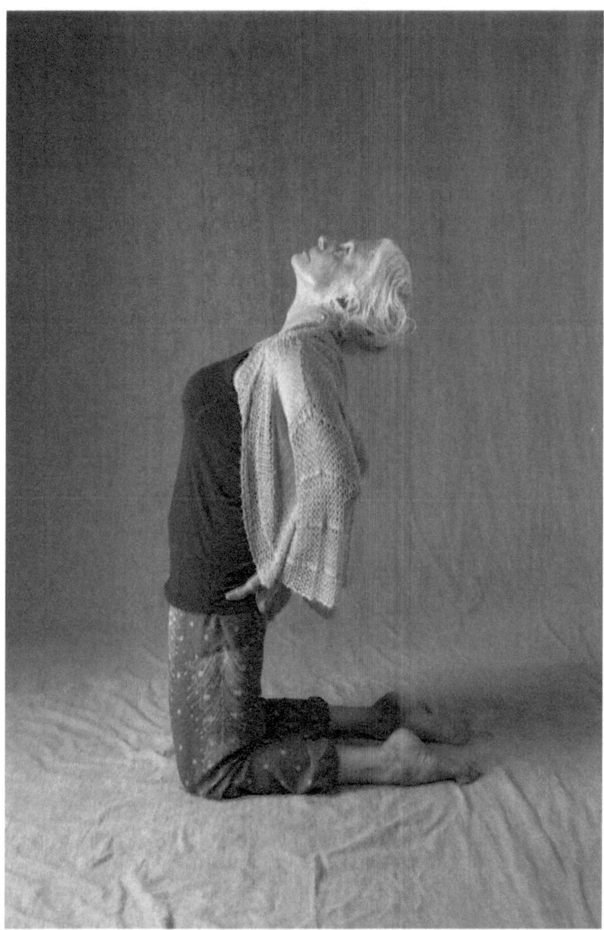

Then reverse the bend by bringing your head back toward your feet. Your hands on your hamstrings will help support this movement. Then straighten out your head so it is aligned with your body. Breathe in with the backward arch; breathe out as you straighten.

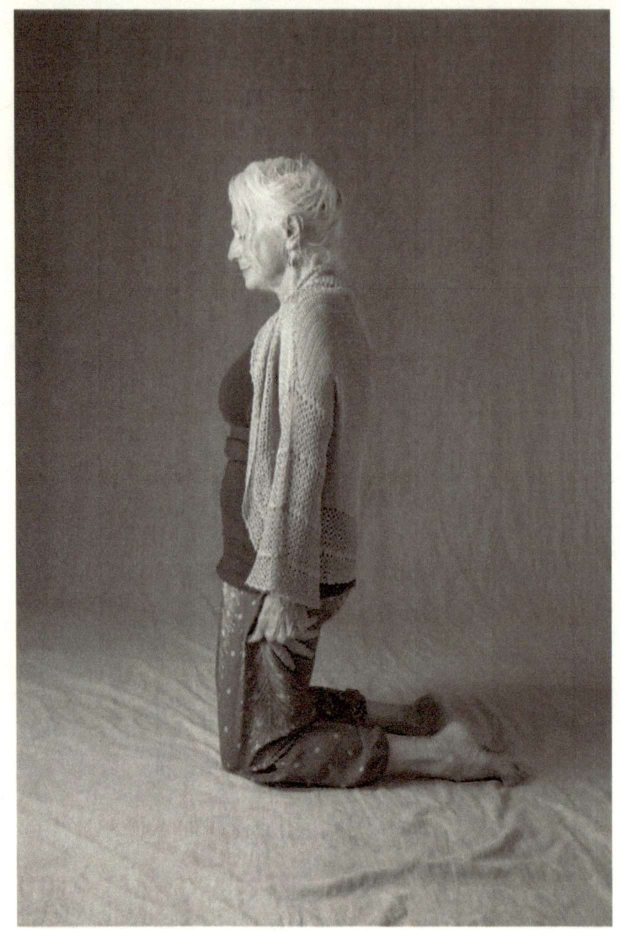

The Fourth Rite

Sit on the floor with your legs straight out and your feet twelve inches apart. Place the palms of your hands on either side of your buttocks. Tuck the chin in toward your chest.

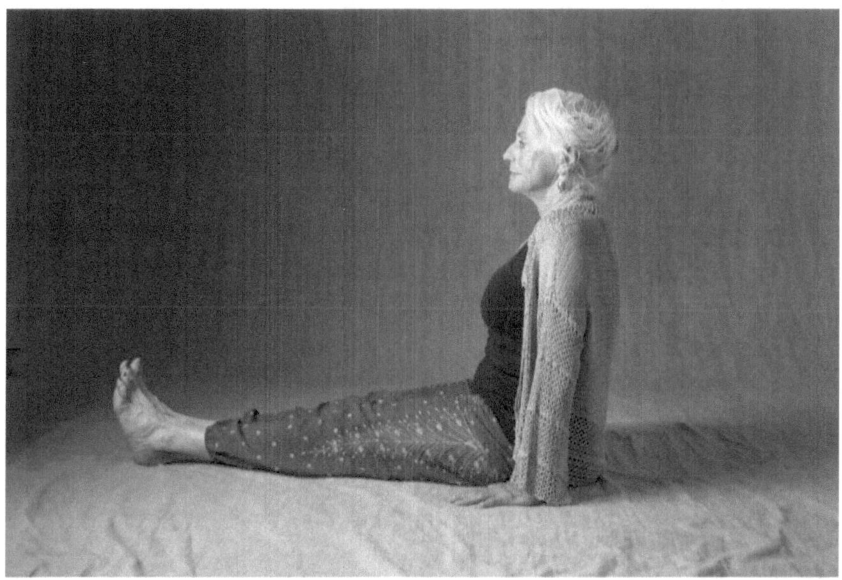

Then drop the head backward while at the same time raising your body and keeping your legs bent.

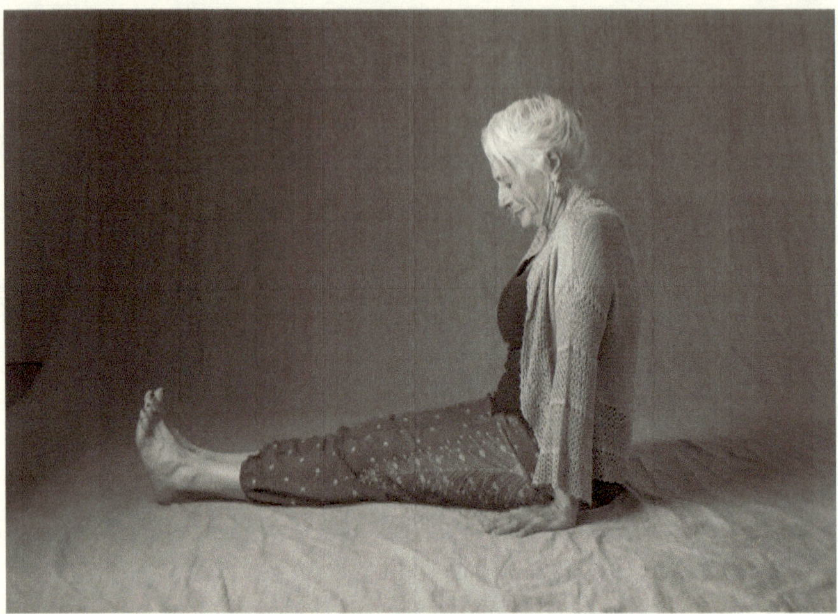

The trunk of the body should be in a straight line with the upper legs. First tense your muscles, and then relax by coming back to the seated position. Breathe in as you lift your body and out as you lower your body. The raised body will resemble a tabletop with the arms and legs representing the four legs of the table.

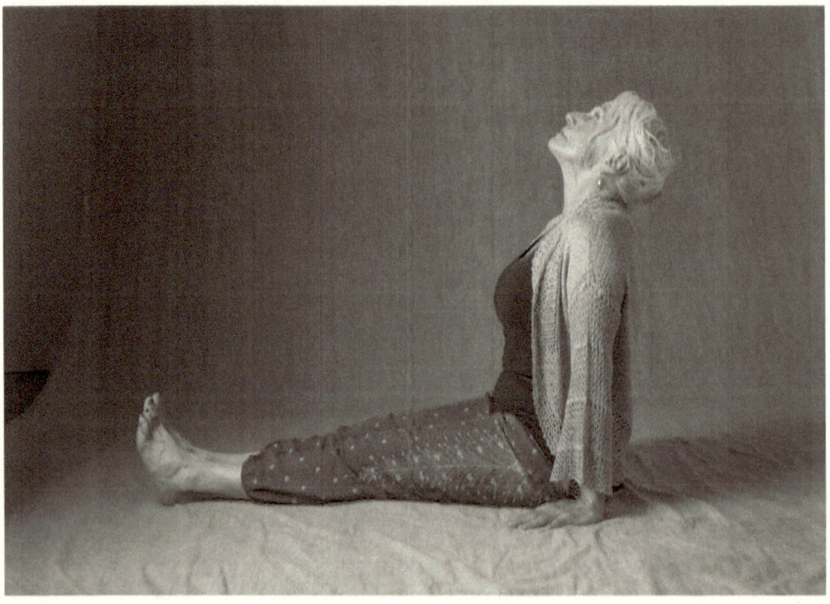

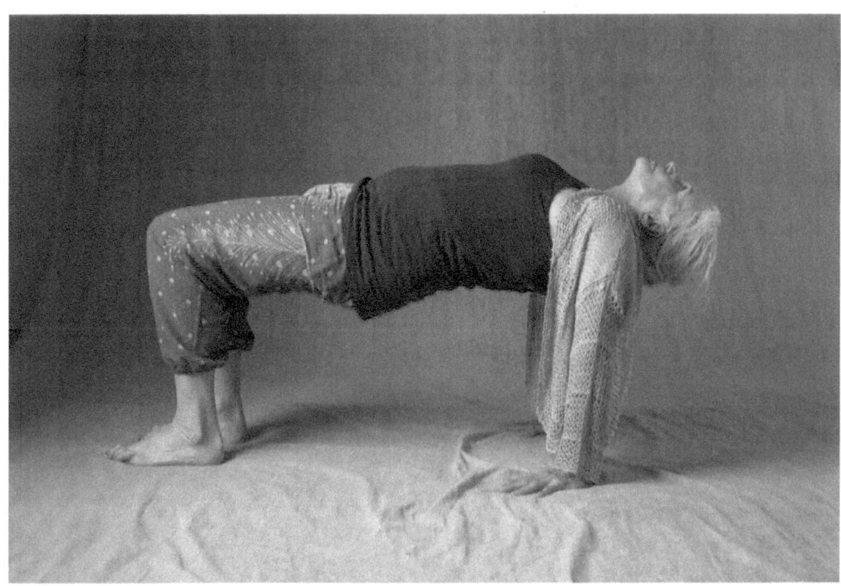

Fifth Rite

Begin with your body face down on the floor. Your arms and legs will support you. The arms and feet should be two feet apart and kept straight. Start perpendicular to the floor, then arch the spine and throw your head back as far as possible.

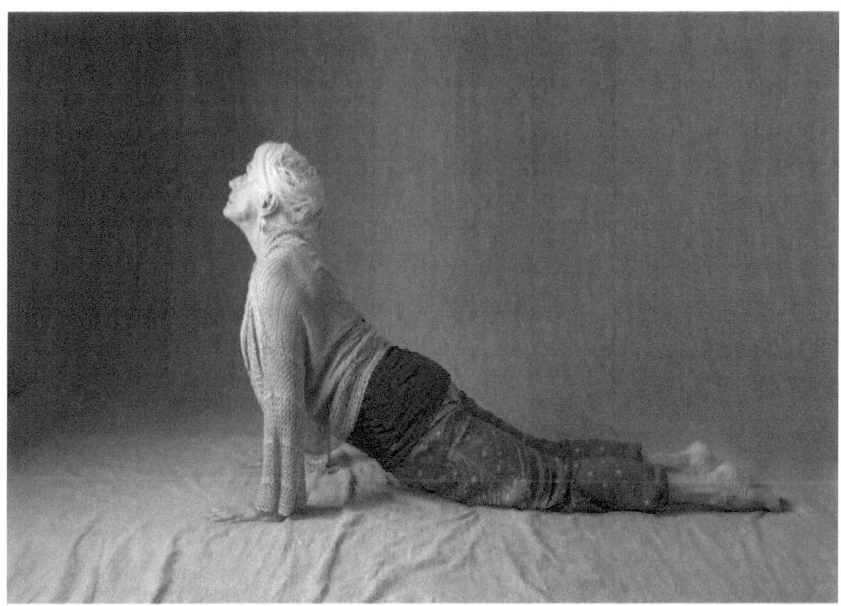

Then bend at the hips and bring your body back, tucking the chin into the chest. This position will resemble an inverted V. Breathe in deeply as you raise the body; breathe out as you lower it.

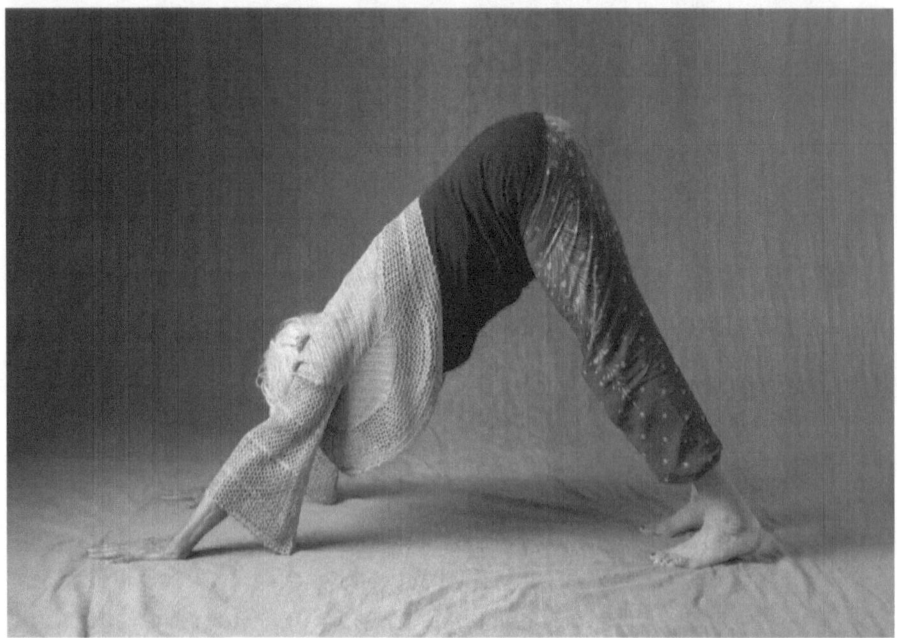

The rites can be done anytime during the day. For best results, it is good to perform them six days a week. You can do a set in the morning, and then again later in the day to build up to the twenty-one. These rites are meant to enhance your entire system, so relax and enjoy. It is suggested not to take a cold bath immediately after the exercises.

Author's note: I have performed these exercises for many years now and find them to be strengthening for my whole body as well as the organs. I also have a tremendous amount of energy during the day.

Healthy Numbers

Dr. Mehmet Oz, director of the Cardiovascular Institute and the Complementary Medicine Program at New York-Presbyterian Hospital and author of over 400 publications and medical books, believes that these eight numbers are important to monitor for better health.

Blood Pressure: aim for 115/75

The average middle-aged person's blood pressure is 130/80, which Dr. Oz says isn't good enough since cardiovascular disease is already a major health problem.

Resting Heart Rate: 83

Before rising, take your pulse by placing two fingers on your carotid artery or wrist. Count beats per minute. If your resting heart rate is higher than eighty-three, Dr. Oz says you are at a higher risk for a heart attack. In order to improve your resting heart rate, it is vital to increase your physical activity. While exercising, subtract your age from 220 and multiple that number by 0.8. The final number will give you your ideal rate.

Cholesterol: 2 to 1

If you have a family history of high blood pressure, diabetes, or if you smoke, your LDL (bad) level should be under one hundred. If you have none of these risk factors, between one hundred and 129 is optimal. Your HDL (good) level should be above sixty. Doctors say the measurement of LDL to HDL should be less than two to one, though a ratio of three to one is still manageable.

Omega-6 to Omega-3s: 4 to 1

Eat more fish, whole grains, ground flaxseeds, beans, and nuts. Limit processed foods and oils from safflower, corn, cottonseed, and peanuts. A balance of omega-6 and 3 will help to decrease risk of cardiovascular disease, certain cancer, arthritis, and asthma.

Inflammation: 1

A blood test can gauge your C-reactive protein (CRP). If your number is under one, your chance of having heart disease is less than half. If the number is above ten, other ailments may be present, which include autoimmune disease. For prevention, floss daily and consume more of the Mediterranean diet to include vegetables, whole grains, olive oil, fruits, and an occasional glass of wine. I cannot help wondering that if this testing had been available during my mother's life, her rheumatoid arthritis may have been managed better and she may have been given a longer life.

Vitamin D: 30

A blood test result should show a hydroxy level between thirty and fifty. During the winter months we are exposed to less sunshine. Deficiencies may lead to multiple sclerosis, cancer, heart disease, and osteoporosis. My mother also suffered from osteoporosis. Perhaps if my mother had heeded my father's wisdom to relocate to the sunny Arizona desert, she would have felt better.

Lack of sunshine and the damp, cold northeastern climate made my mom's physical condition worse. Take a supplement with at least 1,000 milligrams of vitamin D3 or cod liver oil daily. My grown children remember drinking cod liver oil while they were growing up. They still make faces telling me that story.

Blood Sugar: 125

Your blood sugar should register under 100 after an eight hour or overnight fast. If you're not fasting, the number should be less than 125. Eat chia seeds in yogurt or salads; they help slow the rate at which sugar is absorbed.

Bone Density: 1

The standard DEXA 9 dual energy X-ray absorptiometry scan gives your bone density and compares it to that of a young woman. Above one is normal; one to 2.5 indicates osteopenia which could lead to osteoporosis; above 2.5 indicates osteoporosis. This testing is recommended for women who are no longer on hormone replacement therapy. It is generally good to be tested around age fifty for women who have had a family history of osteoporosis or a hip fracture. To help maintain bone strength and density, take a daily dose of 1,000 IU of vitamin D, 1200 milligrams of calcium, and 400 milligrams of magnesium and do strength and resistance training two to three days a week.

Healthier Living Beyond the Challenges

Stanford University's Patient Education Research Center has developed a project called "Healthier Living with Ongoing Health Problems." This program currently is implemented in sixteen states and seventeen countries. One thousand participants were involved in a five-year research project that showed that people who attended the program improved their health behaviors through exercise, cognitive symptom management, coping, and better communication with physicians. They also noticed a decrease in fatigue and distress as well as a significant decline in the duration of hospital stays.

If you are concerned about diabetes, arthritis, heart disease or other chronic health conditions, you might want to consider taking this course. It is also offered online.

The Blue Zones

For five years, Dan Buettner, along with National Geographic, the National Institute on Aging, European demographers, medical scientists, and journalists, researched four regions of the world where people live longer and healthier lives. The survey included lifestyle, diet, medicines, socialization, and physical activity. These places were coined the blue zones. There is a three times better chance of these blue zone cultures becoming centenarians (100 years of age or older) than those who do not live in these four zones.

Loma Linda, California USA

This town contains a large community of Seven Day Adventists. They are a devout group who have a large and supportive community which supports one another culturally and socially.

Seven Day Adventists

Their foods are plant-based from grains and seeds and inspired from the book of Genesis. Saturdays are their Sabbath or what they call the "sanctuary in time." Their life expectancy is nine to eleven years longer than their American counterparts.

Sardinia, Italy

This is the next stop in the fountain of youth tour. Sardinia is an island off the coast of Italy. There are more male centenarians living here than anywhere else in the world.

This sounds like a good life to me. Also, on Sardinia, the elders are greatly respected, a contrast to our culture in America where many elders are forgotten.

Italians

Giovanni Sannai, 104 years old, chops wood and has his morning glass of red wine rich in antioxidants. He beat Buettner in a round of arm wrestling.

Nicoya Peninsula, Costa Rica

The Nicoya Peninsula on the West Coast of Costa Rica is a third blue zone where people live to a ripe old age surpassing one hundred. A traditional day for Panchita, who is deaf and partially blind and celebrated her one-hundredth birthday in 2008, would be rising at 4:00 a.m., praying, gathering up her chicken eggs, grinding corn by hand, making coffee, and gathering her water from the nearby well. Her breakfast meal consists of tortillas, eggs, and beans. She then splits wood and clears bush away from her modest home. Residents grow their own gardens for fresh food. Her son is eighty— a great-grandfather who still exudes plenty of energy. The Nicoyan community is a close-knit group where families live together, have a strong support system among their friends, and display the belief that they will always be taken care of by God no matter what challenges may arise in their lives.

Costa Ricans

They live simply without adding stress to their daily lives. Through a lifestyle passed down from their indigenous roots of the Chorotega, they exhibit a low rate of heart disease and have strong bones and hips, which may be attributed to their drinking water source containing high amounts of calcium.

Okinawa, Japan

The last stop along the road to longevity is Okinawa, the main island off the coast of Japan. This area holds the current world record for life span, with the average age of women at eighty-five and men at seventy-eight years of age. There are over 457 centenarians on Okinawa and most people who live the longest are free of disabilities. Also, the eighty- and ninety-year-olds are as healthy and active as people thirty years younger.

The people of Okinawa have a strong sense of community and family, have healthy habits, and are relatively free of stress, unlike most of the world. Their life purpose, faith, and perhaps their affinity toward mugwort sake may give them healthier years ahead.

Japanese

Their diet consists of several servings of fruits and vegetables each day. Fish is consumed several times a week. They are physically active and involved in numerous activities such as walking, gardening, dancing, and karate, all performed without going to a gym.

Genes may play a 50 percent part in our destiny. However, if we mirror different lifestyle choices that are similarly reflected in the blue zones, such as aging gratefully, gracefully, and healthfully, we can gift ourselves a longer and happier life. This chapter has presented you with oodles of exercise suggestions. It does take discipline and an awareness of our bodies and our health. Even my grandmother, with only one leg, managed to walk each day. Take the steps to physically be the best person you can be, and you will reap huge rewards.

If we could give every individual the right amount of nourishment and exercise, not too little and not too much, we would have found the safest way to health.

—Hippocrates

Step 3

Nutrition: We Are What We Eat

When I prepared meals for my five children, we had at least one meal a day in which we would eat slowly and consciously and say a prayer to give thanks for the food before us, the love between us and the friends around us. Those meals became our sharing time. We didn't rush. Sitting around our dining room table we were together as a family—sharing our day, laughing, and coming together to appreciate one another. As a child, I had Sunday dinners with my grandparents in a similar manner. The meals stretched out for hours while we practically worshipped the Italian cuisine lavishly prepared by my grandmother, aunt, and mother. The food was always prepared fresh and in great abundance with ingredients bought from the local Italian grocery stores. On holidays and special occasions, we had Italian ham (prosciutto) laced over melon slices, antipasto, escarole soup, pasta with homemade marinara sauce, meatballs made from beef, pork, and veal, fresh meats or fowl, cheeses, salads, Italian breads, and always the irresistible Italian desserts served with coffee and anisette and hard cookies to dip into the coffee. The Chianti bottle was passed around the table, and there were bottles of soda for the children. Afterward, the men would rest in the living room while the women cleaned the dishes, and the children ran outside to play.

In 1989, the slow food movement began to counteract fast food and fast life. It is now in thirty-two countries. This nonprofit organization introduces origins of local food and the joy of eating foods from various regions around the world. We were living the slow food movement years before it became the thing to do.

Foods and Your Health

Did you know that the top three diseases in the US—heart disease, cancer, and diabetes—can be directly linked to diet? Almost two-thirds of the population of the United States, and over 1.5 billion of the world's population, is now considered overweight. This is at an all-time high. Three hundred million people worldwide are classified as obese. We know that obesity is a causative factor in many diseases, diabetes among them. One in three children born today will have diabetes in their lifetime.

Alzheimer's disease, which affects over 6.5 million Americans and there are 55 million people affected worldwide, is also impacted by diet. According to a recent study published in the *Annals of Neurology* (2006, vol. 59, no. 6), an emphasis on a Mediterranean diet consisting of fruits, vegetables, whole grains, olive oil, and fish reduced the risks of Alzheimer's. According to a Columbia University study, people who adhered to the Mediterranean diet had a 40 percent lower risk of Alzheimer's than those who did not adhere to the diet.

What we eat is vitally important to both preventing and reversing disease and maintaining our good health. The current health-care system in America does not promote disease prevention, simply because health-care providers are in the business of treating sickness. The pharmaceutical industry, food producers, and restaurants are all in business to make money. It is up to us to decide what is good for us and take responsibility for our overall health. Don't stress about food. Remember, nutrition plays a vital role in our lives. If you overeat, undereat, or feel guilty about what you eat, you won't be doing yourself any favors. So, relax about your intake and know that you will make wiser food choices as your body becomes stronger and leaner.

Paybacks

- Boost metabolism.

  As we continue to age, our metabolism slows down as much as 20 to 40 percent. Metabolic Syndrome makes a person more susceptible to diabetes, heart disease, and strokes. Over forty-seven million Americans have been diagnosed with metabolic syndrome; people who are overweight and obese are more likely to develop the syndrome.

Healthy foods and regular exercise can assist in boosting a sluggish metabolism. Add a variety of fresh fruits, nuts, eggs, vegetables, and fiber to your daily diet. Enrich your diet by including omega-3 foods, salmon, and tuna. Omega-3-rich foods can boost our metabolism to help burn calories.

Avoid processed foods and fast-food restaurants.

- Improve heart health.

  Many people have unhealthy diets filled with saturated fats, including white flour, donuts, cakes, pies, cold cuts, bacon, breaded and fried meats, full fat dairy products, canned fruits, and fried vegetables. The result is a high probability of coronary artery heart disease, high blood cholesterol, and high triglycerides.

  Introduce healthier foods. Monounsaturated fats and polyunsaturated fats can assist in lowering blood cholesterol. Eat low-fat proteins, which include low-fat dairy products, egg whites, skinless chicken, and free-range meat. Include fresh fruits, vegetables, and whole grains, reduce salt consumption, and make food portions smaller.

- Lower cholesterol.

  Cholesterol is a type of fat. In the previous chapter, we have discussed the two types: the "good fat," HDL and the "bad fat," LDL. Triglyceride is also another lipid (fat) which should be monitored. Remember the Duke University Medical Center and East Carolina University study? Overweight people who exercised at least thirty minutes a day were able to lower their LDL. The ones who added more vigorous exercise such as up to twenty miles a week of jogging not only lowered LDL but also increased HDL rates.

Begin by including unsaturated fats: soybean, sesame, and olive oils to name a few. Be wary of commercial dressings which may also contain saturated fats. Egg yolks, some shellfish, high fat dairy products, organ meats, and poultry all contain cholesterol. Vegetables, nuts, seeds, fruits, and grains do not contain cholesterol. Oats, barley, oranges, apples, and beans may help to decrease cholesterol amounts. Plain complex carbohydrate foods like rice, pasta, and potatoes can be included without adding creams or rich sauces.

- Prevent joint pain/arthritis.

People who weigh 20 percent or more than the normal average for their age are more likely to place more stress on knees, hips, legs, spine, and feet. My mother was treated for her rheumatoid arthritis with corticosteroid therapy. There were days her feet were so swollen she couldn't walk. After several years of receiving multiple cortisone shots and gold injections, her hands and feet still became permanent twisted shapes. Arthritis drug side effects may increase appetite, promote weight gain, and produce fluid retention. Osteoarthritis may also contribute to weight gain.

Throughout the years, people with arthritis have complained of joint swelling and pain after consuming eggplant, potatoes, tomatoes, and peppers, all from the nightshade family. Sugar, red meat, chocolate, salt, additives, and preservatives may also be contributing factors. There is little research connected to diet and arthritis. However, eating cold-water fish like salmon, sardines, and trout which contain high levels of omega-3s may aid in reducing inflammation within the body. Drinking three to four cups of green tea (polyphenolic compounds) a day may also help to decrease certain RA symptoms.

- Prevent Alzheimer's.

  Alzheimer's research has been discussed in the "mind" section of this book.

  Nutrition plays an important role in keeping our brains smart and keeping Alzheimer's at bay. Have a healthy, well-balanced diet, limit sugar and salt intake, and drink eight glasses of water a day. Eggs are rich in acetylcholine, a neurotransmitter. Low levels of this have been linked to patients with Alzheimer's. Salads are packed with antioxidants to help ward off free radicals from forming and help provide better cognitive skills. Yogurt contains tyrosine, an amino acid, which helps our memory and alertness. There are complications that arise if a person is in a more aggressive stage of Alzheimer's. When the nerve cells die off, a person may lose interest in food, have difficulty eating, and not recognize whether they are hungry or thirsty. At this stage, medical supervision is vitally important.

- Prevent inflammation.

  Dr. West, referred to in the supplement section, says that inflammation occurs through cell damage and eating wrong foods: sugar, processed, charbroiled, and barbequed foods, pasta, breads, pastries, and baked goods, which can increase levels of pro-inflammatory peptides. Our organs directly benefit from a healthy, anti-inflammatory process.

  Suggestions include vegetables, olive and coconut oil, flax seeds and nuts, and aloe vera juice. Eat fish high in omega-3s twice a week and ingest or cook with olive, hempseed, flax, avocado, rice bran, coconut, or walnut oils. Green, orange, and yellow vegetables, blueberries, spinach, soy milk, and tofu all have anti-inflammatory properties. Avoid cooking or using canola, corn, cottonseed, safflower, sunflower, rice bran, and soy oil.

- Prevent diabetes.

  Over thirty-four million people in America have been diagnosed with diabetes. Worldwide the statistics are at 422 million people. That number will rise by the year 2025 to 385 million people, making the disease a worldwide epidemic. Over 100 million people in America have been diagnosed with Type 1 diabeties. Type 1 diabetes occurs among younger people and is commonly treated with insulin injections. Type 2, which affects 90 percent of those diagnosed with diabetes, occurs after age forty and can often be treated through exercise, diet, and medication.

  If you have been diagnosed with diabetes, ask yourself, "What foods help to control my blood sugar, blood pressure, and help keep cholesterol levels in a healthy range?"

  Maintaining a diet which contains 70 percent alkalized foods helps keep the pH levels healthy. Dark green leafy vegetables and salads assist in helping rid the body of acid-forming chemicals. Limit unhealthy fats, sugary sweets, and add to your diet more fiber and low glycemic foods, which consist of protein, low glycemic carbohydrates, and omega-3 foods. A low glycemic plan helps to keep energy high during exercise, maintains healthy weight ad healthy cholesterol levels, and increases insulin resistance. There are charts on the internet which list low glycemic foods.

My Kitchen Secrets

I preface this section to share my latest nutritional habits. Know that it's good to listen to your body when it is about nutritionally healthy foods for you.

I do not eat twelve to sixteen hours after my last evening meal. Intermittent fasting has given me a new lease on life. I feel more energized and focused. I usually only eat two meals daily now. I am eliminating as much dairy as I can. I avoid sugar. To determine how much sugar is in a product, look at the label and reduce the carbohydrate amount by the fiber amount. Don't pay attention to the sugar amount on the label.

At one time or another I have joined an organic co-op to stock my kitchen with local vegetables and fruits. I was a vegetarian for many years; however, because I am physically active and live at a higher altitude, I made the change to eat high-quality protein. I eat very little red meat, but when I do it's organic, and usually buffalo or elk. I only eat organic fowl. I eat cold-water fish such as halibut or salmon twice a week. Usually, I have smaller portions of protein mixed with larger portions of vegetables. Basically, I purchase locally grown pesticide-free or organic fruits, vegetables, grains, nuts, and fish. I focus on keeping my diet 80 percent alkaline and 20 percent acid. If the body becomes too acidic, health issues can arise. I encourage you to purchase Shelley Young's recipe books. The meals are simple and good and will help familiarize you with eating alkalized foods.

Breakfast

I will eat a small serving of buckwheat, oatmeal, or quinoa, adding a small amount of raw almond butter which is ground in my Vitamix, slivers of apple, banana, strawberries, or blueberries, and ground flaxseed. I include walnuts, which are high in essential fatty acids, or raw almonds which I soak in water and place in a jar in my refrigerator, making them more digestible. Consume the nuts within two days. Eating complex carbohydrates an hour before a workout or class is very beneficial. It provides energy. For sweeteners, I use a packet of stevia which is a natural sweetener and safe for diabetics. The more alkaline the body becomes, the more the craving for donuts, breads, sweets, and processed foods disappears. If I am headed to an exercise class, I take a bottle of water and add a teaspoon of powdered greens and vitamin C. This drink is packed with protein, enzymes, and amino acids, and keeps me hydrated.

Late Morning Post-Workout

I prepare a protein meal which helps rebuild muscle I have spent during my workout routine. I am not a fan of protein bars, although I understand their concept if you are participating in a run or bike race or other high-energy activities. I concentrate on feeding my body with organic healthy sources which include farm fresh eggs, organic, unsweetened non-dairy yogurt or a protein drink with lecithin, banana, blueberries, and flax oil.

Lunch

This is a great time for me to get my live (not cooked) foods. I make a large salad of organic greens, dark leafy vegetables, carrots, avocado, celery, cucumbers, sprouts, pumpkin seeds, add a small amount of cold-water fish such as trout, salmon, sardines or cod. This is my high-protein meal in the middle of the day when my metabolism is high, and my system can easily digest the food. My energy level stays satisfied until dinner.

Mid-Afternoon Snack

Raw nuts such as almonds, hazelnuts, pecans, pistachios, pumpkin, and sunflower are especially nutritious and alkaline. It's a good idea to soak these nuts, which helps to activate the enzymes, making them easier to digest and increasing the nutritional value. Cover nuts with water and refrigerate the container for an hour (overnight for almonds). Rinse and eat within two days to prevent mold from forming.

Another treat could be an Ezekiel™ tortilla, which you can find in many health food and grocery stores in the refrigerator section. Mash up an avocado with tomatoes and spread on the tortilla.

Dinner

This meal should be eaten at least three hours before bedtime. Our metabolism slows down as we approach the end of the day, so in order to digest food properly, do not eat too late in the evening. The adage "Eat like a king in the morning, a queen in the afternoon, and a prince in the evening" does contain powerful wisdom.

I enjoy warming foods at this time: vegetable soups, or lightly steamed vegetables. Before bed, I prepare herbal tea sprinkled with cinnamon, and I sleep like a princess without the pea.

Eating Tips

When diet is wrong, medicine is of no use. When diet is correct, medicine is of no need.

—Ayurvedic Saying

If your kitchen has been stocked with fresh, whole foods, you are well on your way to vibrant health. Your body and mind will be happier for feeding it well. Food which is locally grown and free of pesticides and sprays should always be your number one choice. I like to prepare my produce when I bring it home by washing it, cutting it and placing it in refrigerated containers. I do not refrigerate my tomatoes and some of the bananas get peeled and go into a freezer bag. I use them for my protein drinks. Here are several tips for healthy eating:

- Eat whole foods that have not been chemically sprayed, and always rinse your produce with a fruit/vegetable product which removes any remaining chemicals and sprays.
- Avoid corn syrup, food colorings, monosodium glutamate, and other artificial additives.
- Season with garlic, turmeric, kelp, seaweed, cinnamon, cayenne pepper, and sesame seeds.
- Avoid sugar, too much caffeine, and any processed foods.

- Avoid getting your carbohydrates from refined foods high in sugar; eat only complex carbohydrates.

- Indulge in raw and lightly steamed vegetables, tofu, small quantities of cold-water fish (twice weekly), garlic, fresh grains, legumes, nuts and seeds, sprouts, tomatoes, avocados, lemons, limes and grapefruit, and at least sixty ounces of purified water a day. Greens contain more than enough to meet the body's protein requirements (elephants and gorillas eat only grass and leaves and look at their strength); eating hot peppers can relieve cluster, migraine, and sinus headaches.

- Buy free-range, organic meat or fowl only; you will be consuming a product free of hormones, arsenic, or antibiotics.

- Consume foods that contain antioxidants, including leafy greens, broccoli, spinach, kale, nuts, apples, blueberries, cherries, grapes, and even Spirulina, all of which support the body, ward off senility, and fuel the brain. Our brains contain high levels of fat; when we eat the wrong kinds of food, free radicals attach to the fat.

- Eat small meals during the day, eat only when hungry, and slowly chew your food. This can help keep our metabolism charged and keep the pounds off. The Centers for Disease Control recommends 1,600 calories a day for women and 1,900 for men. According to *The Journal of the American Medical Association* (*JAMA*), cutting down on daily food intake can extend your life.

- Eat locally grown foods that are in season. When I was living in Hawaii, seasons were very subtle, but I still found myself eating warming soups and more grains and proteins during the winter months when the temperatures were lower. In the spring, add greens, berries, and sprouts, and in the summer months, eat more fresh vegetables, greens, carbohydrates, and fruits, which help to detoxify the body and supply needed energy.

- Have your main meal in the middle of the day; your muscles are strong in the morning, but in the middle of the day, your digestion is strongest.
- Eat breakfast, lunch, and dinner, and eat sensibly for your weight and size.
- Eat slowly in a quiet, tension-free environment.
- Avoid snacking or grazing during the day, especially on sugar and simple carbohydrates such as chips.
- Avoid trendy diets that may initially appear to be working but eventually become more detrimental to your physical balance, producing fatigue, stress, depression, and high acidity which will cause your weight to yo-yo.
- Slow down; when we eat on the run, we usually down empty calories and deny our bodies wholesome nutritional antioxidant packed foods.

Should My Food Be Cooked or Raw?

I feel better when I eat 70 to 80 percent raw or lightly steamed foods. I also like to lightly steam vegetables to go along with my salad. Too much cooked food slows my digestion and makes me feel sluggish. Dr. Gabriel Cousens recommends taking a B12 supplement if you don't eat animal protein.

Paybacks of Eating Live Food

- Lower cholesterol and triglycerides.
- Lower incidences of stomach cancer.

- Build a stronger immune system.

Some foods retain more of their nutrients when cooked, such as cabbage and tomatoes, although grains and beans are more acidic when cooked. If your diet consists mainly of cooked foods, you can slowly introduce raw or live food to your meals. For instance, at lunch time, have a salad along with your protein source. Eventually you will begin to eliminate cooked foods and find yourself eating carrot or celery sticks dipped in guacamole. Your system will become more alkaline and your cravings for gooey processed foods and sweets will be greatly diminished. You will be sending different "messages" to your body and over time it will become part of your lifestyle.

Results of Cooking Food

When we heat food over 114 degrees, it destroys live enzymes and destroys up to 80 percent of vitamins and minerals. According to Gabriel Cousens, MD, we lose more than 90 percent of a food's B12, half of the protein, and one hundred percent of enzymes and phytonutrients.

We are presented with various ways of eating. There's diet after diet program. Many stay around for a while, and others drift away. I am mentioning some of the programs that have stayed around and seem to be talked about on podcasts, social media, and websites. I feel it's important to determine if any of these programs benefit you, especially if you are overweight, older, or under a doctor's care.

Paleo

This diet refers back to the caveman days and suggests that people incorporate the same kinds of foods that go way back. A modern paleo diet includes fruits, vegetables, lean meats, fish, eggs, nuts, and seeds. These foods were commonly gathered and consumed thousands of years ago. The belief is that we should consume foods that are connected to our gene pools rather than foods connected to modern day farming methods. Farming introduced dairy, grains, and legumes.

Pros

- To assist in weight loss.
- To help cardiovascular disease.
- To decrease blood pressure.
- To lower cholesterol and triglycerides.

Cons

- Lack of fiber through whole grains, legumes, and low fat dairy.
- Lack of nutrients, vitamins, minerals, protein, and calcium.
- Costs more.
- Not enough long-term studies.

What to Eat

A modern Paleo diet includes:

- Fruits.
- Vegetables.
- Nuts and seeds.
- Eggs.
- Lean meats, especially grass-fed animals or wild game.
- Fish, especially those rich in Omega-3 fatty acids, such as salmon, mackerel, and albacore tuna.
- Oils from fruits and nuts, such as olive oil or walnut oil.

This information comes from the Mayo Clinic (mayoclinic.org)

Keto Diet

This diet restricts carbohydrates, starches, fiber, and sugar to less than 50 grams a day. When carbohydrates are consumed, energy is activated in the cells; however, the energy lowers, which increases the appetite. When fats and proteins are consumed, digestion slows down and hunger takes longer to produce. Carbohydrates store water in the body. On Keto, water is not stored, which is why it's important to stay hydrated to avoid kidney stones.

Some foods consumed are meat, fish, avocados, and high-fat dairy items. Grocery stores are providing more Keto friendly choices.

Pros

- Helps to lose weight.
- Lowers cardiovascular risk factors.
- Helps to manage insulin levels.

Cons

- Food cost higher.
- May cause headaches, bad breath, and constipation.
- Strictness of diet may make it difficult to stay on.

Mayo Clinic Diet

The Mayo Clinic Diet has less saturated fat and includes extra-virgin olive oil, avocado, salmon, nuts and seeds, berries, beans, and carb-containing veggies.

Safe Cookware

- Ceramic enameled cookware has good heat distribution, is dishwasher friendly, and is easy to clean and maintain.
- Copper cookware is lined with tin or stainless steel to keep

copper from getting into foods and the pots have even heat distribution, but keeping copper pots shined is a task.

- Stainless steel cookware is made up of small amounts of different metals and is safe to cook with.
- Aluminum cookware is now anodized, which makes it safe and nonstick and scratch resistant; this is my current choice.
- Teflon cookware is relatively safe, and the Environmental Protection Agency (EPA) says the small Teflon flaking doesn't affect our health; if you are unsure about Teflon, do some research.
- Cast iron pots and pans are excellent to have in your kitchen; they need to be seasoned and washed without soap; I used mine for years at home and while camping.

Water

How much pure water do you consume each day? How pure is your water source? If you are not a "water person," or if you wait to drink water when you are thirsty, chances are you are already in a state of dehydration. If you exercise and sweat or live in a humid climate which causes you to perspire, and you do not drink adequate amounts of water, chances are you are very dehydrated.

A good rule of thumb is to drink at least sixty-four ounces of good water daily. Better yet, drink ten to twelve, eight-ounce glasses daily. As we've mentioned, soft drinks and caffeinated beverages will dehydrate our bodies. Many of us fill up on soda, juice, teas, and alcoholic beverages, so we don't have room for pure water. Maybe we don't like the taste of water by itself and want to add something to it to make it more palatable. It's important that we break ourselves of this habit and learn to love the taste of pure water.

On the flip side, too much water can be dangerous as well. Athletes who constantly drink large amounts of water can experience a condition called hyponatremia, where salt levels in the blood fall dangerously low. That's why it's important to consume electrolytes if you are exercising, running, or working out and consuming large quantities of water.

What Is Safe Drinking Water?

During the 1990s my publishing company, Kali Press, came out with a book titled *Don't Drink the Water (without reading this book): The Essential Guide to Our Contaminated Drinking Water and What You Can Do About It* by Lono A'o. The book lists the health hazards involved in drinking public as well as groundwater. It highlights the many contaminants that are put into our public water systems and the chemicals being dumped into the soil which then leach into the groundwater. We also see more contaminants such as gas leaks, pesticides, and pharmaceutical drugs leaching into the soil and eventually into the groundwater. Such is the case in California where high levels of TCE contamination have become a major health hazard in certain areas. California is not alone in this epidemic. Stronger standards need to be enforced on local, state, and federal levels. Besides a link to cancer and the nervous system, contaminants also can disrupt our hormonal balance. This is not a pretty picture.

Although I am not a trained scientist, my research throughout the years has led me to understand that certain public water systems, untested wells, living around chemical plants or large industrial complexes and certain bodies of water all may be contributing factors in our poor health. Meanwhile, what can you do to obtain better drinking water? The bottled water industry has exploded. It seems every time you go to the supermarket there is another brand of bottled drinking water on the shelf. Now we can choose between spring water, distilled water, natural artesian water, mountain spring water, alpine spring water, and many more to add to the confusion. Bottled water doesn't have to comply with stringent testing guidelines, so what you think you are drinking may not necessarily be the best water.

It's also a good idea to drink water from glass or stainless containers. Drinking water from a plastic bottle which has been exposed to high heat (perhaps while in your car) is not advisable as certain toxins from the plastics can leach into the water. Various plastics leach a chemical called bisphenol A (BPA) which mimic female hormone estrogen. In the USA over 90 percent of Americans age six and up have experienced higher levels of BPA, which may lead to obesity, infertility, and some forms of cancer. Avoid plastic bottles which have the number three, six, and seven on the bottom and consider purchasing stainless bottles. Kleankanteen.com sells 100 percent recycled food grade stainless drinking containers for adults and children.

Choosing a Water Filter

In order to filter out harmful substances in your water, you can test your water for chlorine, lead, mercury, aluminum, cadmium, chromium, copper, bacteria, viruses, and radioactive material such as radon and uranium. There are filtration systems which range in choices from pitchers to countertop, under sink purifiers, and full house systems. Don't forget to research shower and tub filters while you are at it. The skin is our largest organ, after all, and absorbs everything. I have a water filter at my kitchen sink and a shower filter to eliminate public water additives. I have a large crock pot with a spigot in which I store my drinking water.

Patrick Flanagan

"Don't over medicate—hydrate!"

Patrick Flanagan has been touted as a unique, mature, and inquisitive scientist featured in the 1962 Life Magazine edition. At eleven years of age, he developed a guided missile detector which the US military bought. Throughout the years, Flanagan has been instrumental in developing books, products, and devices based on water. One of his products is called "Crystal Energy" which, when added to water, increases the water flow and nutrients through the cell membranes to nearly two and a half times faster than ordinary water. This mixture of aqueous blend of silica and other salts assists in cell hydration. The benefits of Crystal Energy are:

- Silica to support detoxification.
- Enhanced circulation healthy cell growth.

I put ten drops in eight ounces of purified water and drink it three times daily. I live in a high-altitude climate, which can make you dehydrated. I have discovered that I require less water during the day because I am not as thirsty. This product has been available for over forty years and holds several patents.
This information comes from www.phisciences.com.

First-Rate Fats

We have become a low- and no-fat society, but this is not particularly healthy. Eating fats that do not clog the arteries is the key to getting proper nutritional values from fats. About 20 percent of your diet should be made up of healthy fats. What are some of those good fats?

- Polyunsaturated fats such as evening primrose, flaxseed, grape seed, and borage are all available in capsules or gel caps. These fats help the body eliminate acids, regulate hormones, and develop healthy cells.
- Monounsaturated fats include olive oil, raw nuts, and

avocados; these fats increase your energy and contribute to healthy, vibrant skin.

- Essential fatty acids—these are the good fats which the body achieves through your diet; they are long-chain polyunsaturated acids which include omega-3, 6, and 9. Essential fatty acids are necessary to elevate mood, provide beautiful skin, increase a healthy immune system, support mental clarity, and normalize weight (you need to eat fat to burn fat). They produce prostaglandins which support healthy heart function, blood pressure, and blood clotting.

Brands—Uses and Storage

Some brands recommended for supplemental oils are Udo's Choice®, Barlean's Organic Oils®, and Omega Nutrition®, all available in health food stores and food markets.

Do not heat these oils. Add them to salads, smoothies, or to cooked vegetables. Store your oils in a place away from heat after opening.

Benefits of Flax:

Lignans provide up to 700 times the amount of fiber found in legumes or whole grains which help prevent certain cancers.

One tablespoon of flaxseed oil will provide the daily amount of linolenic acid. Whole flaxseed can be put in a grinder. Store it in a sealed glass container in your refrigerator. Use it in smoothies, protein drinks, on cereal and in plain yogurt. Flaxseed can be sprinkled on any food.

Paybacks

- Rich in omega-3s and lignans which are natural antioxidants.
- Helps prevent heart disease.
- Helps remove toxins.

- Helps allergies and digestive problems.
- Provides healthy skin, hair, and nails.
- Better brain development.
- More rapid healing.
- Improves athletic performance.

Coconut Oil

Coconut oil contains high levels of lauric acid, which makes it an excellent preventive for heart disease. Its antiviral, anti-fungal, anti-microbial, and anti-tumor properties lower blood cholesterol and arterial plaque as well as strengthen the immune system. Coconut oil also stimulates metabolism and activates normal thyroid function, which does decline with age. It contains medium-chain fatty acids, which are more easily digested and metabolized in the body. I cook with coconut oil. It has a high smoke point of 350 degrees replacing many oils including olive oil. Olive oil is great uncooked as in a salad dressing or drizzled over vegetables. I purchase high-quality organic coconut oil. It keeps forever without refrigeration. It is a great substitute for people who have nut allergies. Your body will love three and a half tablespoons of coconut oil per day (melt and consume), or you can drink ten ounces of coconut milk to get the same benefit.

Coconut Oil Suggestions

- Popcorn: add two tablespoons of coconut oil and a quarter cup of popcorn kernels to a pan over medium to high heat; cover, shake the pan to evenly distribute the kernels.
- Oatmeal: stir one tablespoon into hot oatmeal and sprinkle with cinnamon.
- Smoothie: add one tablespoon into soy or almond milk; add one frozen banana, blueberries, and blend.

Recipes

Veggie—Flax Burgers

1 6.5 ounce jar artichoke hearts, drained and quartered

1 teaspoon chopped garlic

¼ cup chopped green onions

3 tablespoons chopped fresh parsley, or 2 teaspoons dried

¾ cup cooked garbanzo beans, drained and rinsed

¾ cup cooked kidney bean or black beans, drained and rinsed

3 tablespoons ground flaxseed, regular or golden

2 tablespoons roasted tahini or other nut butter

4 generous twists of black pepper

½ cup cooked brown rice or millet

Cooking spray

4 whole grain hamburger buns (optional)

Place artichoke hearts, garlic, green onions, parsley, garbanzo beans, kidney or black beans, ground flaxseed, sesame tahini, and pepper in a food processor; pulse about eight times, until blended. Scrape down sides and pulse another six times. Do not overprocess. Transfer to a bowl and gently stir in cooked rice or millet. Divide mixture into four portions and form into patties half-inch thick. Heat a large, nonstick frying pan over medium heat and coat with cooking spray. Fry burgers until bottoms are brown, about five minutes. Spray tops of burgers with cooking spray and flip. Cook until brown, about five minutes. Serve on buns if desired.

Per serving: 215 cal., 37% fat cal., 9g fat, 1g sat. fat.,10g protein, 24g carb., 9g fiber, 331 mg sodium.

I have made these burgers many times and found them yummy and a terrific substitute for a meat burger. You can use lean meat like buffalo or elk if you have meat eaters in your family. This recipe has protein, fiber, and the benefits of healthy fats. Try it with lettuce, sliced tomato, and avocado.

Avocados

Avocados contain 10 to 15 percent protein and little sugar (about 2 percent). They are loaded with minerals, including iron, copper, and more potassium than bananas (which are high in sugar). They contain a high-quality fat which quickly satisfies hunger. Eating avocados improves your red blood cells, and the lutein in avocados helps to protect against cancer and eye diseases.

I eat at least one avocado a day, although two or three are very beneficial and will not make you put on extra weight. Do not combine them with proteins or melons.

Avocado—Sprout Salad

2 cups sprouts

½ cup diced celery

½ cup diced red onion

½ cup thinly sliced carrots

1 red pepper, diced

4 teaspoons lemon juice

2 teaspoons dulse flakes

1-2 avocados

In a small bowl, combine the sprouts, celery, onion, carrots, red pepper, lemon juice, and dulse. Toss thoroughly. Add the avocados and mix gently. Serve on a lettuce leaf. Serves two. *Recipe from* The Raw Gourmet *by Nomi Shannon.*

Goat Cheese

For people who are lactose intolerant, goat cheese is a great substitute for regular cheese, making it more tolerable and digestible. It is also lower in fat and calorie content. It provides a great source of calcium, boosts metabolism, is easy to digest, and is high in protein. It contains potassium, vitamin A, selenium, niacin, and tryptophan. One of my granddaughters is lactose intolerant; however, she can digest goat's milk and cheese. I enjoy it sprinkled in salads and in an appetizer spread in lieu of cream cheese. Try it on pizzas and in pasta dishes.

Other Healthy Foods to Consider

Quinoa

Quinoa, once a staple food of the Inca civilization, is now considered the super grain. It is a complete protein and provides all eight essential amino acids as well as minerals, B vitamins, and fiber. Quinoa can be purchased at any health food store, specialty food store, and some grocery chains. I enjoy eating it warm, but it also makes a delightful cold salad. Here is one of my favorite recipes for quinoa:

Plum Quinoa Salad

Preparation 20 minutes, cooking time 12 to 15 minutes, chilling time 1 ½ hours.

1¼ cups quinoa

2½ cups water

2 large ripe plums, pitted and diced

½ cup chopped, toasted walnuts

¼ cup chopped red bell pepper

¼ cup chopped yellow bell pepper

¼ cup sliced green onions

2 tablespoons flax oil

3 tablespoons extra-virgin olive oil

¼ cup white wine vinegar

1 ½ tablespoon of stevia or natural cane sugar

¼ teaspoon sea salt

Rinse quinoa and drain well. Add to boiling water; reduce heat, and simmer covered for twelve minutes. Remove from heat and let stand for five minutes. Fluff with fork and let chill for about thirty minutes. Stir together quinoa, plums, walnuts, peppers, and onions in a medium bowl. Whisk together oils, sugar, and salt in a small bowl and pour over salad; toss well to coat all ingredients with dressing. Cover and chill for one hour. Makes six servings.

Nutrition information per serving; 370 cal., 23g fat (2g saturated), 0g chol., 100mg sodium, 36g carbohydrates, 4g fiber, 8g protein.

This is such a nutritious salad, and very tasty, too. Plums are rich in antioxidants and contain iron, potassium, and vitamin E; flaxseed oil contains essential fatty acids and B vitamins; and walnuts are heart healthy with high amounts of omega-3 fatty acids.

Sun-Dried Tomatoes

These tomatoes contain lycopene which is a photochemical and antioxidant that fights free radicals in the body. Sun-dried tomatoes contain twelve times the amount of lycopene compared to a regular tomato. They are a good fat, low in salt content, calories, and fat, and contain no cholesterol. Sun-dried tomatoes are best when mixed with olive oil. They can be used in salads, chicken dishes, and eggplant or pasta dishes.

Sardines

The name comes from Sardinia, a small island off the coast of Italy. Sardines contain high levels of omega-3s, which assist in lowering triglyceride levels. Sardines are a great anti-inflammatory. They also are high in vitamin D, calcium, B12, selenium, protein, and contain three times the amount of phosphorus than milk, spinach, and bananas. They also contain coenzyme Q10 (CoQ10), a nutrient found in cells which has antioxidant and immune system properties. I buy wild sardines in olive oil. I eat them plain or mixed into salads.

Greens

All foods and supplements give off an electrical charge; fresh green live food contains higher frequencies than cooked, processed foods. Dr. Maximilian Bircher-Benner, a scientific researcher, states "The absorption and organization of sunlight, the essence of life, is derived almost exclusively through plants. Since light is the driving force of every cell in our bodies, that is why we need green plants."

Robert O. Young, PhD, a world-renowned microbiologist and nutritionist, heads up the InnerLight Biological Research Center in California. His research in the last twenty years has led to a new biology of eating, which includes green alkaline foods.

Green food includes grasses and greens; key ingredients being organic wheat grass, barley, and kamut grass. Irish moss helps to bind mycotoxins and flush them out of the body. Green powder is also an excellent source of protein. Drinking two to three liters a day of green food mixed with pure filtered water also serves as your water quota (usually one-half of your body weight in ounces of water). If you weigh 150 lb., you would take in seventy-five ounces of water daily. Water intake is vital to maintain healthy, vibrant skin and bathe your blood cells to halt dehydration.

Green foods also assist in shifting our blood cells and tissues from acid to alkaline. Dr. Young's studies have shown that the blood pH level affects every cell in our bodies. As we change from acid to alkaline, disease cannot exist, weight normalizes, depression lifts, and our quality of life is greatly enhanced. The goal here is to consume 80 percent alkaline foods or beverages. It's simple to check your acid-alkaline levels using pH strips available at pharmacies. The ideal blood pH is 7.365. Testing first thing in the morning is best.

I had considered my diet healthy until I changed to Dr. Young's suggested food groups while in my fifties. I discovered, for instance, that my breakfast of fruit and yogurt was on the acidic side. I started drinking two 32 oz. bottles of green drink daily for a couple of weeks and gradually increased it to three to four 32 oz. bottles. I noticed almost immediately that my joints began to ache as my body gradually released the acid buildup. For me, it began with my feet and traveled up my body to my head.

Cleansing Power Drinks

Today, I make a blended drink with rice or soy milk, protein powder, super greens, avocado, liquid lecithin, and Udo's Choice® Oil Blend, which contains omega 3-6-9 essential fatty acids. Upon rising, I drink a glass of warm water with a squeeze of lemon or lime juice, and sometimes I add a pinch of cayenne pepper. This combination balances the pH, provides excellent energy, and is a great morning cleanser.

Juicing

It is difficult to eat four to five servings of vegetables and fruit in one's daily diet. Juice provides a complete compliment of vitamins, minerals, and enzymes which nourish your body and improve your health. Drinking two glasses of fresh juice daily along with a balanced diet can give you boundless energy and sometimes reverse long-term illnesses.

I have two juicers: a Vitamix® and a Juiceman®. The Vitamix is pricey but practical. It doubles as a blender to make smoothies and soups as well as juicing vegetables and fruits.

Because I live in the mountains, I tend to eat more warming foods during the winter months; however, come early spring I begin to reintroduce raw foods and juice back into my daily diet. Explore the numerous juicers available and you will discover it is a worthwhile kitchen appliance which serves you well. I encourage you to use fresh farm grown organic ingredients. Juicing will provide fiber to keep you regular and help prevent colorectal cancer. Do not take the easy road by purchasing bottled juices. Often, they have preservatives and are heated for pasteurization. They're definitely not fresh, so any nutrients are lost. Keep in mind to remove apple seeds, remove skins from grapefruits and oranges, and eliminate the greens from carrots as they can be toxic.

Drink Your Greens: Paybacks

- Lowers blood pressure.
- Improves skin, hair, and nails.
- Prevents arthritis.
- Improves eczema.
- Increases metabolic rate to help with weight loss.
- Normalizes fat metabolism which may decrease insulin dependency.
- Kills cancer cells.

Green Tea

There are a variety of different green teas available in the market; Genmaicha is a Japanese tea which is a favorite among adults as well as children. Bancha contains calcium, vitamin A, niacin, and iron. There are many Chinese green teas. I always brew my green tea with care. I do not pour boiling water on the tea leaves and only brew for two to three minutes. A longer steeping period will make the tea bitter tasting.

Paybacks

- Helps retard tooth decay because of its natural fluoride.
- Helps with gastrointestinal disorders.
- Eases hemorrhoids.
- Lowers high blood pressure.

- Lowers fever.
- Promotes urination.
- Eases headaches.
- Helps control dizziness.
- Dilates blood vessels.
- Helps prevent blood clots.
- Reduces cholesterol.
- Is a powerful antioxidant as well.
- Burns calories and helps with weight loss.

I also recommend white, black, and herbal teas.

Miso

Miso has friendly bacteria, with essential amino acids, digestive enzymes, vitamins, and absorbable protein. Miso is made up of fermented soybeans and koji. It is important to obtain the unpasteurized version from the store and preferably a product that has been fermented for at least 180 days.

Miso Benefits

Many studies have been done on miso, some on humans and some on animals. These studies are showing the following benefits of miso:

- Reduces risks of cancer, including breast cancer, prostate cancer, lung cancer, and colon cancer.
- Protects from radiation.
- Immune strengthening.
- Antiviral—miso is very alkalizing and strengthening to the immune system helping to combat a viral infection.

- Prevents aging—high in antioxidants, miso protects from free radicals that cause signs of aging.
- Helps maintain nutritional balance—full of nutrients, beneficial bacteria, and enzymes, miso provides protein, vitamin B12, vitamin B2, vitamin E, vitamin K, tryptophan, choline, dietary fiber, linoleic acid, and lecithin.
- Helps preserve beautiful skin—miso contains linoleic acid, an essential fatty acid that helps your skin stay soft and free of pigments.
- Helps reduce menopausal complaints—the isoflavones in miso have been shown to reduce hot flashes.

Miso Soup Recipe

5-inch strip wakame (sea vegetable)

1 large onion (about 1 cup)

4 cups filtered water

2 tablespoons miso (ideally, fermented for 6 months–2 years)

Garnish—chopped parsley, green onions, ginger, or watercress

Instructions

- Soak the wakame in water for 10 minutes and slice it into 1.5 inch pieces.
- Thinly slice onions.
- Put water, onions, and wakame in a saucepan and bring to a boil.
- Reduce the heat to simmer for 10–20 minutes, until tender.
- Remove 1.5 cups of broth from the saucepan, place in a bowl. Allow water in the bowl to cool a bit and add the miso, mixing it into the water (the water should not be

boiling, because it can kill the live beneficial microflora and enzymes in miso. In general, the microflora in koji, the starter used to make miso, die at 105° F).

- Turn off heat, allow the water to cool a bit.
- Add the miso broth to the soup in the saucepan and add chopped parsley, green onions, ginger, or watercress for garnish.

This information comes from www.bodyecology.com.

Turmeric

This is a plant which is also known as curcumin. There have been over 7,000 studies on turmeric with little side effects. I take a supplement one to two times daily and in the evening make a "Golden Milk." Recipe is below.

Benefits of Turmeric

- Anti-inflammatory managers.
- Prevents rheumatoid arthritis.
- Lowers blood sugar.
- Boosts antioxidant levels.
- Kills cancer cells.
- Reduces skin redness and irritations.
- Improves oxygen levels in the brain.

Golden Milk

Heat 1/2 cup of purified water and add 1/4 cup of organic turmeric powder. Stir for 7-8 minutes. This will thicken. Add a sprinkle of black pepper and a small amount of sesame oil or Udo's Choice®. If mixture becomes too thick, add a small amount of water. The final product should be a paste. Refrigerate in a glass container.

This should last up to three weeks. Heat milk—coconut, almond, rice, organic milk, or soy. Add 1 teaspoon of the paste and stir. You may add raw honey to sweeten. Drink in the evening. Enjoy!

Bone Broth

Generations before made bone broth for their families. This mineral rich broth boosts the immune system and improves digestion. It is excellent for bone and tooth health and contains magnesium, calcium, and phosphorus. The broth has a high collagen content which improves joints, hair, skin, and nails. In addition, the broth contains two amino acids. This first is glycine, which helps digestion and regulates blood sugar levels. It also helps to regulate human growth hormone. It improves memory and reduces stress. The second is proline, another amino acid that helps to reduce blockages in the heart and blood vessels.

Preparing Bone Broth

It is vitally important to obtain meat and poultry from the highest quality sources available—grass-fed beef, organic poultry, and wild fish.

Bone Broth Recipe

2 pounds (or more) of bones from a healthy source

2 chicken feet for extra gelatin (optional)

1 onion

1 carrot

2 stalks of celery

2 tablespoons apple cider vinegar

Optional: 1 bunch of parsley, 1 tablespoon or more of sea salt, 1 teaspoon peppercorns, additional herbs or spices to taste. I also add two cloves of garlic for the last thirty minutes of cooking.

You'll also need a large stock pot to cook the broth in and a strainer to remove the pieces when it is done. Aim for 2 pounds of bones per gallon of water. This usually works out to 2-3 full chicken carcasses.

You'll also need some organic vegetables for flavor. These are actually optional but add extra flavor and nutrition. Typically, I add (per gallon of water and 2 pounds of bones):

1 onion

1 large carrot (if from an organic source, you can rough chop and don't need to peel)

2 celery stalks, rough chopped

If you are using raw bones, especially beef bones, it improves flavor to roast them in the oven first. I place them in a roasting pan and roast for thirty minutes at 350.

Then, place the bones in a large stock pot (I use a 5-gallon pot). Pour (filtered) water over the bones and add the vinegar. Let sit for 20-30 minutes in the cool water. The acid helps make the nutrients in the bones more available.

Rough chop and add the vegetables (except the parsley and garlic, if using) to the pot. Add any salt, pepper, spices, or herbs, if using.

Now, bring the broth to a boil. Once it has reached a vigorous boil, reduce to a simmer and simmer until done. These are the times I simmer for:

- Beef broth/stock: 48 hours
- Chicken or poultry broth/stock: 24 hours
- Fish broth: 8 hours

During the first few hours of simmering, you'll need to remove the impurities that float to the surface. A frothy/foamy layer will form, and it can be easily scooped off with a big spoon. Throw this part away. I typically check it every twenty minutes for the first two hours to remove this. Grass-fed and healthy animals will produce much less of this than conventional animals.

During the last thirty minutes, add the garlic and parsley, if using.

Remove from heat and let cool slightly. Strain using a fine metal strainer to remove all the bits of bone and vegetable. When cool enough, store in a gallon size glass jar in the fridge for up to five days or freeze for later use.

Homemade broth/stock can be used as the liquid in making soups, stews, gravies, sauces, and reductions. It can also be used to sauté or roast vegetables.

Especially in the fall and winter, we try to drink at least one cup per person per day as a health boost. My favorite way is to heat eight to sixteen ounces with a little salt and sometimes whisk in an egg until cooked (makes a soup like egg-drop soup) (wellnessmama.com).

German Tonic

I make this simple formula when I feel lower in energy or during spring and fall detox time.

Paybacks

- Immune booster.
- Liver cleanse.
- Prevention of infections and colds.
- Prevention and treatment of clogged arteries.

Recipe

4 organic lemons with peels

4 large garlic heads

1 small organic ginger root

2 liters of purified water

- Wash lemons and cut into small pieces. Peel garlic and add with ginger to blender and blend ingredients together.

- Heat 2 liters of water (8 cups) and add blended ingredients, do not boil. Remove just before boiling point. Let mixture cool and strain ingredients store in glass container in refrigerator.
- Drink one cup two hours before meals. Be sure to shake the glass bottle well.

What to Avoid or Minimize

Before I sound like a preacher, I want to remind you that life is meant to be enjoyed. I am not suggesting you stop eating everything you enjoy but am asking you to take a look at how often and how much you are eating certain foods and beverages that may be detrimental to your health and well-being over a period of time. Balance, after all, plays a vital role in our day-to-day world.

Corn Syrup

I challenge you to find a traditional food or beverage product that doesn't contain high fructose corn syrup. In a study published in January 2009 in the scientific journal, *Environmental Health,* mercury was found in nearly 50 percent of tested samples of commercial high fructose corn syrup. The news is disturbing given that this ingredient is present in a large portion of processed American foods. According to David Wallinga, MD, coauthor of the study, "Given how much high fructose corn syrup is consumed by children, it could be a significant additional source of mercury never before considered. We are calling for immediate changes by industry and the FDA to help stop this avoidable mercury contamination of the food supply." A separate study by the Institute for Agriculture and Trade Policy detected mercury in nearly one-third of fifty-five popular brand-name food and beverage products where high fructose corn syrup is the first or second highest labeled ingredient, including products by Quaker®, Hershey's®, Kraft®, and Smuckers®.

Sugar

Sugar consumption in the US in 2003 averaged 120 lb. per person per year. Americans typically use twenty teaspoons of sugar per day. Cutting that consumption in half would help to eliminate excess sugar in our diets. Prior to the turn of the last century (1887-1890), the average sugar consumption was only five lb. per person per year. Cardiovascular disease and cancer were virtually unknown in the early 1900s; do you think there is a connection? Sugar has been shown to cause inflammation in our bodies, and attaches to collagen, resulting in stiff, inflexible, sagging skin, and is the most aging food for your body and skin. Controlling our blood sugar level and insulin levels will not only improve our overall health, but give us beautiful, youthful skin.

Sugar can lead to an overgrowth of yeast in our stomachs. If you have been diagnosed with candida, your practitioner will suggest a simple diet without the sugar. Eat several small meals a day and include protein to assist in diminishing your sweet cravings.

Sugar's Side Effects Include:

- Suppressed immune system
- Hypoglycemia
- Coronary heart disease
- Periodontal disease
- Speeds the aging process, causing wrinkles
- Weight gain and obesity
- Depression
- Kidney damage
- High triglycerides
- High-density cholesterol (HDLs)

- Depletes minerals
- Osteoporosis
- Increases blood platelet adhesiveness, which may result in blood clots and stroke
- Headaches and migraines

Sugar the Natural Way

The FDA has approved Xylitol® (zy-leh-tal) as a sweetener; it is derived from birch—it is not fructose. The World Health Organization has evaluated such Xylitol® products as gum, toothpaste, and candies that may prevent tooth decay. It may also help with periodontal disease and strengthen tooth enamel. Xylitol® products are available at your local grocery and health food stores.

Stevia® (asteraceae) is a member of the sunflower family. It is also labeled in the marketplace as Sweetleaf®. Stevia® contains certain nutrients and can be used by diabetics as it does not contain blood glucose.

Carbohydrates

Carbohydrates, protein, and fats make up the macronutrients in our diets that provide all our calories. Carbohydrates provide most of the energy needed in our daily lives, both for normal body functions such as heartbeat, breathing, digestion, and for exercise such as cycling, walking, and running.

Many people are confused about the differences between simple and complex carbohydrates, and many popular diet books seem to make it more confusing. Carbohydrates are simple or complex based upon their chemical structure. Both types contain four calories per gram. Both are digested into blood sugars called glucose, which is then used to fuel our bodies for work or exercise. The difference is simple carbohydrates are digested quickly. Many simple carbohydrates contain refined sugars and few essential vitamins and minerals. Examples include fruits, fruit juice, milk, yogurt, honey, molasses and sugar, white flour, breads, pasta, and potatoes.

Complex carbohydrates take longer to digest, but also make a lot of acid when they break down. Thus, it is best to limit total carbohydrates to 20 percent of your diet. Feel free to eat broccoli, asparagus, squash, cauliflower, dark greens, celery, cucumbers, sea vegetables, parsley, peas, onions, cabbage, and red, yellow, and green peppers. These vegetables are usually packed with fiber, vitamins, and minerals. Go easy, however, on carrots, beets, and winter squash as they have high sugar content. Avoid, or limit to 20 percent of your diet, corn, wheat, and rice. Add more spelt, buckwheat, quinoa, and millet. These are high in protein, low in acid, non-mucus forming, and help balance sugar levels in the body.

Chocolate

Not all chocolate bars are created equal. Premium Dagoba® bars (available in health food and gourmet stores) contain only four grams of sugar compared to Hershey's Healthy Special Dark Chocolate® which yields twenty-one grams—more than five times as much sugar. Check the sugar content on the chocolate you purchase and remember that dark chocolate contains many more benefits (antioxidants, for one) than milk chocolate. The higher the content is of cocoa, the better. Dark chocolate is a natural antidepressant.

Caffeine

We are a coffee-drinking world. Whether we are sitting at an Italian café sipping an espresso or enjoying a cup of latte at a coffee shop, the tradition of coffee goes way back. Questions have arisen about whether caffeine is healthy for you. However, in recent years it has been found that coffee can cause dehydration, insomnia, anxiety, increased blood pressure, increased urination, and even diarrhea. It can also increase the risk of osteoporosis.

Is drinking four or more cups daily beneficial for you? One study involving 83,000 American women in their mid-fifties who had never had a stroke, diabetes, or heart disease brought surprising results. Two to three cups of coffee a day lowered the risk of stroke by 19 percent. Women who were nonsmokers who drank four or more cups a day reduced the risk of strokes even more to a whopping 43 percent. It may be a little-known fact that twice as many women die from strokes than breast cancer. People who have high blood pressure, insomnia, and other related health issues should always consult with their health practitioner before becoming a coffee aficionado.

I am an occasional coffee drinker; usually organic beans and I enjoy a great cup of espresso. I do suggest, however, if you enjoy coffee, that you purchase organic beans which have not been sprayed with pesticides. When you brew your coffee, use unbleached filters to avoid chlorine leaching into your coffee. Coffee is still acidic (as are sodas), so you may consider switching to herbal teas or black, green, or white teas which are packed with antioxidants. Caffeinated teas contain only 90 mg of caffeine compared to 160 mg in coffee. If caffeine is a problem for you, there are many non-caffeinated teas to choose from. Even if a study originates from a professional peer review journal, common sense and moderation can go a long way.

Saturated Fats

Vegetable oils, when heated, form trans-fatty acids and affect our liver's ability to metabolize properly. Serum cholesterol increases and is deposited on the artery walls. LDL (bad) cholesterol levels rise, which could lead to arteriosclerosis, heart disease, and diabetes. Some of the oils to avoid are canola, corn, soy, and sunflower. These polyunsaturated oils have been shown to contribute to heart disease and weaken the immune system. Canola oil derivative is rapeseed, part of the mustard plant family. Rapeseed, or canola oil as it is commonly known, is used as a lubricant, fuel, and soap, so why would one wish to include it as a food? There are many good oils to cook with and to flavor your salads. Avocado oil has a high heat factor (525 degrees) to cook with. It doesn't burn food as easily as safflower, sunflower, and canola, which have a heat temperature of 225 degrees.

Here are examples of other oils and their heat factors to consider when cooking.

- Almond oil, 495°F
- Corn oil, 450°F
- Peanut oil, 450°F
- Cottonseed oil, 420°F
- Macadamia nut oil, 410°F
- Sesame seed oil (light), 410°F
- Olive oil, 410°F
- Grape seed oil, 400°F
- Walnut oil, 400°F
- Coconut oil, 350°F

Graham Kerr, the Galloping Gourmet®, has forsaken the high fat meals he prepared on his popular television show. His wife and business partner, Treena, discovered that eating rich foods contributed to their seasickness while sailing 24,000 miles on their seventy-one-foot sailboat. In 1981, Treena suffered a stroke and heart attack. Her cholesterol level was at 350. Today she is healthier, and her cholesterol is in a safe range.

While we are on the subject of saturated fats, I recently viewed the documentary *Super Size Me*, directed by Morgan Spurlock and released in May 2004. This film received rave reviews at the Sundance Movie Festival and rightly so. The movie addresses how the fast-food industry promotes unhealthy foods and obesity among young and old alike. It follows Spurlock to McDonald's®, where he ate three regular meals a day for one month. He had a physical exam performed by three doctors before, during, and after the thirty-day period. During the thirty days of his McDonald's® diet, his weight ballooned by thirty pounds, his cholesterol count went up sixty-five points, and his blood pressure went from a normal range to high. After the documentary previewed, McDonald's eliminated their supersize promotions. Just so you know: McDonald's Chief Executive, Jim Cantalupo, died from a massive heart attack and CEO Charlie Bell underwent cancer surgery. Enough said. Grandparents who are concerned about the fast food their grandchildren consume need to see this movie.

Carbonated Soda

Sodas contain phosphoric acid, which interferes with the production of calcium, can create weaker bones, and may lead to osteoporosis. Soda also neutralizes stomach acid which aids in digestion. The sugar content equates to ten teaspoons per drink. Ingredients include caffeine, artificial additives, and high calories. Health effects include high blood pressure, cholesterol, and weight gain.

More No-No's

- Alcoholic beverages
- Chlorinated water
- Microwaved foods
- MSG
- Junk and processed foods
- French fries, unless they are baked and preferably sweet potatoes
- Potato chips: try the organic ones, and watch sodium content and added ingredients
- Fried and grilled foods—gas grills only

- Salt, sea salt okay
- Cured and pickled foods
- Mushrooms (however, certain mushrooms such as maitake and shitake are advocated for cancer prevention and treatment)
- Peanuts: peanuts can cause an allergic reaction, and non-organic peanuts are heavily sprayed and may be susceptible to carcinogenic mold spores; an exception to the peanut rule might be Arrowhead Mills® or other organic peanut butter
- Yeast: a gluten test will determine if you are gluten sensitive; if so, eat gluten-free products

Food Toxins

Fluoride

Even though most western European countries have banned fluoride altogether, Americans ingest it daily through their public drinking water, toothpaste, dental products, beverages, and processed foods. Fluoride has been in the US water supply for over fifty years. The fluoride debate has been going on for many years between the ADA (American Dental Association)—which has strong lobbyists in Washington—and independent scientists who have been researching the effects of fluoride for the last ten years.

As early as 1950, fluoride was given rousing approval by the US Public Health Service, which approved of adding it to American drinking water as it was thought to help in the prevention of cavities. Over 60 percent of the public water in the US now contains fluoride.

The fluoride which is currently used originates from an industrial grade hexafluorosilicic acid used in the air-pollution scrubbing systems of the super phosphate industry. The EPA will not permit this substance to be dumped into the oceans but permits it in our drinking water. Fluoride is as toxic as lead and arsenic and contains small amounts of both elements. Some of the ill effects of ingesting fluoride include:

- Brittle bones and increased risk of fractures
- Compromised tooth enamel
- Higher levels of aluminum and lead in the brain and blood
- Compromised immune system, which can cause the body to attack its own tissue, which may result in tumor growth acceleration

Avoiding Heavy Metals

We have poisoned and continue to poison our environment with cigarette smoke, automobile exhaust, chemical fertilizers, industrial waste, herbicides, and pesticides, to name just a few. Our bodies are in constant battle with these heavy toxins, lowering our immune responses and making us susceptible to illnesses and disease. Mercury, in the form of amalgam (silver) fillings in our mouths, has been linked to multiple sclerosis and other autoimmune diseases.

Consider having your amalgams replaced with composite fillings. I chose to have my amalgams removed while in my forties. A simple test can determine the levels of heavy metals in your body; if they are high, you might want to look into chelation therapy, which can be performed intravenously to remove metals.

There are products on the market that claim to release metals from your body. One product that appears to have studies behind it is zeolite. Make sure you research the products you choose before consumption.

To battle heavy metal toxins in your body, monitor your intake of certain fish. Noted below are some fish to avoid.

- High POPs (persistent organic pollutants): Farmed salmon, limit to once a month if pregnant/nursing

- High mercury: Atlantic halibut, king mackerel, oysters (Gulf Coast), pike, sea bass, shark, swordfish, tilefish (golden snapper), tuna (steaks and canned albacore)
- Moderate mercury: Alaskan halibut, black cod, blue (Gulf Coast), crab, cod, Dungeness crab, Eastern oysters, mahi mahi, blue mussels, pollock, and tuna (canned light)
- Low mercury but overfished: Atlantic cod, Atlantic flounder, Atlantic sole, Chilean sea bass, monkfish, orange roughy, shrimp, and snapper; these sea creatures should be avoided for the environment's sake

Mercury

I eat fish twice a week. I have always been aware that some fish contain high levels of mercury, but I didn't know how much. After some online research (see the end of this chapter for some good websites), I discovered that four ounces of yellow fin tuna (Ahi) provides 90 percent of the maximum weekly limit of mercury. I also found that twelve ounces of crab yields 50 percent of the maximum weekly mercury levels, but twelve ounces of wild Pacific salmon yields only 10 percent.

The *Chicago Tribune* investigated mercury levels in canned fish and discovered that albacore tuna contains three times the mercury level of chunk light tuna! However, several types of tuna may be blended together, so read your labels. I eat a tuna product from Wild Planet® which is lowest in mercury and is sustainably caught.

Blue Marlin, caught in the Gulf of Mexico, polluted by toxic metals and chemicals dumped into the Gulf of Mexico, can contain twenty to thirty times the acceptable levels of mercury. And the disastrous 2009 BP Gulf of Mexico oil spill dramatically changes the picture on whether or not any fish from that area is safe to eat.

There are fish that are lower in mercury and safer to eat, including anchovies, arctic char, crawfish, Pacific flounder, herring, king crab, sand dabs, scallops, Pacific sole, farmed tilapia, wild Alaska and Pacific salmon, farmed catfish, clams, striped bass, and sturgeon. Wild Alaska and California salmon (fresh or canned) are also low in POPs.

Dioxins

Dr. Edward Fujimoto, wellness program director at Castle Hospital, Kailua, Hawaii, says that heating our foods in plastic containers—especially foods that contain fats—releases dioxin, a poison shown to cause breast cancer. Dr. Fujimoto instead recommends using Corning Ware® and/or glass or ceramic containers to heat food in the microwave. He doesn't recommend microwaving TV dinners, instant ramen soups or anything in a paper container. He also believes plastic wraps are dangerous when covered over food heated in the microwave.

Since Dr. Fujimoto's research came out, however, there have been reports that his claims about the release of dioxins are incorrect. The information cited on the internet states that plastic wraps and containers do not contain the chemical components that can form dioxins. Also, this site says that in order for dioxins to be released, temperatures would have to be above 700 degrees Fahrenheit.

My personal view on this controversy is to err on the safe side. I will continue using glass containers as advised by Dr. Fujimoto and do further research on this subject. Until proven otherwise, I recommend:

- Do not use plastic containers or plastic wrap in microwave.
- Do not put your water bottles in the freezer.
- Cover foods in the microwave with glass, ceramic, a paper towel, or parchment paper.

Pesticides

Dr. Andrew Weil has stated that environmental toxins can create diseases. However, manufacturers of pesticides have told us that there is no conclusive evidence that there is any harm in eating produce and fruits which have been sprayed with pesticides. What are we to believe? We know that long-term exposure to pesticides can affect the endocrine, hormone, immune, and nervous systems. Pesticides have also been linked to cancer, reproductive problems, and neurological disorders, and can be especially harmful to the elderly and anyone suffering from a deficient immune system.

I buy organic produce whenever I can and wash my fruits and vegetables with a vegetable and fruit wash which can be purchased at any grocery store. Many fruits and vegetables (grapes, apples, cucumbers, etc.) are coated with a wax, so you'll need to scrub all that off. There are a variety of produce washes in the market such as Veggie Wash®, which claims it safely and effectively removes wax, soil, and agricultural chemicals found on standard and organic produce.

Artificial Sweeteners

Two professors at Purdue University have discovered that artificial sweeteners block the part of you that senses when you're getting full. In other words, they disarm your body's first defense against obesity. Their results, published in the *International Journal of Obesity*, showed that "mouth feel" plays a crucial role in the body's ability to sense the number of calories that are being consumed—and that artificial sweeteners disrupt the natural calorie "count" based on sweetness.

There Are Several Artificial Sweeteners in the Marketplace.

- Splenda® is also known as sucralose, which is the newest artificial sweetener to hit the marketplace. It is 600 times sweeter than regular sucrose (table sugar) and converts from cane sugar to a no calorie chemical sweetener. Chlorine is one of the most dangerous chemicals in sucralose. Side effects can include hives, nausea, diarrhea, heart palpitations, and depression. Most short-term studies have been done on animals, with few human studies conducted.

- Aspartame was approved by the Food and Drug Administration in 1981. It is now included in 6,000 food products. It goes by several trade names: NutraSweet®, Equal®, and Sugar Twin®. The studies done on the side effects of aspartame have been conflictive. H.J. Roberts, MD, has written a book citing the side effects of ingesting aspartame. Some of these side effects are headaches, abdominal pain, dizziness, anxiety, tinnitus, and vomiting.

- Saccharin is the oldest member of the family. It has been available for one hundred years. It is known as Sweet and Low®, Sweet N Low®, Sweet Twin®, and Necta Sweet®. A study done in 1977 showed bladder tumors in rats after ingesting saccharin. Rather than removing the product from production and sale, a warning was placed on the product. There were over thirty more studies done and in 2000, the National Institute of Health Toxicology Program determined that the 1977 study had high dosages of saccharine and more recent studies showed saccharine to be safe and free of carcinogens. People who have allergic reactions to sulfa may experience dizziness, headaches, diarrhea, and shortness of breath.

Due to conflicting studies and reports, it is advisable to research studies on ingesting artificial sweeteners and consider alternatives such as stevia.

Sulfites

I am a label reader and have been for many years. When my children were small, we would go food shopping together to get them in the habit of reading labels on boxes, cans, and frozen foods. One ingredient which appeared over and over was "sulfites." Sulfites appear on labels as sulfur dioxide, potassium bisulfite or potassium metabisulfite, sodium sulfite, sodium bisulfite, and sodium metabisulfite. Sulfites supposedly act as preservatives, decrease bacteria growth, and provide longer shelf life—all beneficial to the food industry. However, it's safe to eat products that don't contain sulfites; if you suffer from migraine headaches and food sensitivities, you may want to consider avoiding them.

Some foods that commonly contain sulfites are wine (both red and white), beer, shrimp (fresh and frozen), canned vegetables and fruit, dried fruit, trail mix, potato chips, molasses, condiments, pickled foods, and vegetable juices. Also, bacon and ham and processed meats contain sulfites. Who knew so many products contain sulfites. Read the labels in your health food store and grocery store to find products that are sulfite-free.

MSG

Have you noticed that some Chinese menus say "we will omit MSG upon request"? What exactly is MSG (monosodium glutamate)? It is a chemical that seems to be in everything: canned soups, chips, ramen noodles, boxed hamburger mixes, canned gravy, many frozen prepared meals, and salad dressings, especially the healthy, low-fat ones. Don't be fooled by an ingredient called "hydrolyzed vegetable protein," either. That is just another name for monosodium glutamate. Check your labels.

So why could this chemical be so bad for you? Studies have shown that MSG can be addicting, and that foods containing MSG can cause overeating and obesity. Some people also have an allergic reaction to it. Fast-food chains such as Burger King®, McDonald's®, Wendy's®, TacoBell® and restaurants like TGI Friday's®, Chili's®, Applebee's® and Denny's® use MSG in abundance.

Years back, I would pick up chicken for my family at Kentucky Fried Chicken® and consume the breaded skin like crazy before I even got home. To my disbelief, I now realize that the crust was coated with MSG. I cringe when I hear the latest commercials for KFC® tout that their chicken now is trans fat free. That may be well and good; however, I question whether it still contains MSG and if their chickens are free-range and fed a healthy diet.

Is MSG a preservative or a vitamin? It may be neither according to John Erb. In his book *The Slow Poisoning of America*, he wrote an exposé of the food additive industry in which he states that "MSG is added to food primarily for the addictive effect it has on the human body" (Erb and Erb, 2003).

Food and Health Conditions

Age Spots

Older people's skin often develops brown spots on the face and hands. Consider exercising several times a week, limiting excess sun exposure and adding a healthy diet. Dandelion tea helps to cleanse the liver, and going on a cleansing diet twice a year, in spring and fall, helps to lighten the spots. Juice or eat carrot, kale, parsley, spinach, green peppers, grapefruit, and lemons.

Aging

This book has discussed nutrition, exercise, supplements, and reduction of stress as examples that are extremely beneficial to help slow down the aging cycle. When juicing or eating, consider deep green leafy vegetables such as kale, broccoli, and spinach—all excellent sources of vitamin C, E, selenium, and beta-carotene.

Alzheimer's Disease (Presenile Dementia)

Remember when cooking in aluminum pots was the norm? Now we have a variety of other cooking options which include ceramic and stainless steel. However, there are many products still in the marketplace which contain unhealthy levels of aluminum. These include deodorants, drink containers, antacids, buffered aspirin, certain toothpastes, shampoo, and baking powder.

By avoiding aluminum products, you can help to halt the buildup of heavy medals in your body, which may prevent a future possibility of getting this disease. Eating sulfur-rich foods helps to cleanse your body of heavy metals. Eating sardines and salmon helps to produce coenzyme Q10, an antioxidant which assists in providing more oxygen in your cells. Juice or eat carrot, kale, parsley, spinach, oranges, and grapefruit, which supply beta-carotene, vitamin C, and bioflavonoids.

Osteoarthritis (OA)

This degenerative joint disease is typically characterized by the thin layer of cartilage between the joints which gradually erodes and wears away. As the protective layer of cartilage vanishes, the bone beneath becomes pitted and uneven, and the structural integrity of the joint is destroyed. Movement can become extremely painful and, in the worst cases, people who have severe osteoarthritis can no longer take care of themselves on a day-to-day basis. There are five stages of OA. Although there is no specific cause, risk factors can include obesity, age, and muscle weakness of the large muscles around the knee. Physical therapy, knee braces, and surgery are some treatments to alleviate OA. Beta-carotene is an antioxidant which is found in many foods: spinach, kale, romaine lettuce, pumpkin, cantaloupe, peppers, and carrots.

Rheumatoid Arthritis (RA)

Connective tissues and joints in hands and feet may lead to deformities. Juicing wasn't popular in the middle of the twentieth century when my mother was ill with RA. Looking back on my mother's diet and weight, I have surmised that by eliminating certain foods and adding others, she may have been able to eliminate many of her chronic symptoms, which included pain, swelling of her feet and crippling of her hands, and prevention of future diseases, which included lupus. My mom ate certain foods that are from the nightshade family. These include tomatoes, eggplant, peppers, and potatoes, all of which my mother prepared and were served often at our meals. These vegetables are known to inhibit collagen repair to joints and produce inflammation and degeneration. Certain citrus fruits also have similar reactions: grapefruit, lemons, limes, and oranges. Foods that contain omega-3s, fatty fish, fruits, vegetables, grains, and legumes may make symptoms less severe. Juice or eat dark leafy vegetables like kale, broccoli, parsley, and spinach, which provide excellent sources of vitamin C and pantothenic acid. Add olive oil and soy products. Carrots, ginger root, and apples increase copper intake. (I remember my mom wearing a copper bracelet.) Pineapple contains bromelain, which helps with digestion, while cherries and blueberries are excellent sources of bioflavonoids.

Atherosclerosis

Hardening of the arteries is a condition which affects millions of people worldwide. Diet and exercise play a huge part in prevention. Avoid caffeine, hydrogenated oils, and alcohol. Juice or eat kale, spinach, parsley, carrots, ginger root, and garlic, which are all beneficial for helping to reduce cholesterol and formation of blood clots.

Cataracts

There are many causes of cataracts: a gradual loss of vision, disease, ultraviolet light, radiation, injury, and aging. Consultation with an ophthalmologist is advised if you suspect or develop cataracts. To help prevent or delay cataracts, the supplement bilberry helps by removing chemicals from the retina of the eye. It is also high in bioflavonoids. Avoid direct exposure to the sun by wearing sunglasses coated with a UVA and UVB lens. Juice or eat parsley, spinach, garlic, broccoli, orange, ginger root, and beet greens, which are all excellent sources of vitamin B, E, C, and beta-carotene.

Diabetes

Eat a high fiber, whole grain diet with oats, barley, and beans along with a good assortment of vegetables and protein. Have citrus fruits and berries, nuts, avocados, olive oil, fish, poultry, eggs, and reduced fat dairy products. Obtain a list of foods that are low glycemic foods. Avoid saturated fats and eat small, frequent meals to keep your weight in a healthy range.

Heart Disease

High cholesterol, diabetes type 2, and obesity are conditions that can lead to heart disease. Foods that support a healthy heart include fruits and whole grains, beans, legumes, nuts, vegetables, potatoes, peas, low-fat breads, cereal, rice, and pasta. These are low in cholesterol and fat. Avoid baked goods and dishes with cream sauces. Avoid deep fried foods, duck, goose, organ meats, cold cuts, and saturated fats. Eat six ounces of protein daily. This includes fish twice a week, excluding lobster or shrimp. Eat skim or low-fat dairy products. Do not eat fats which include butter, ice creams, and sour cream. Limit healthy oils in salads and cooking to eight teaspoons a day.

Inflammation

Inflammation is the basis of many age-related diseases, such as heart disease, diabetes, breast and prostate cancer, autoimmune disease, asthma, allergies, arthritis, deteriorating mental ability, and wrinkled, sagging skin. Dr. Samuel West, who has studied the lymph system for many years, claims that healthy cells contain just the right amount of fluid around them without creating any fluid pressure. The blood maintains the fluid pressure by means of blood proteins—albumin, globulin, and fibrinogen. It enhances normal cell growth and joint mobility. Inflammation occurs any time a cell is damaged through trauma, injury, toxins from bites, waste products from our metabolism, or microorganisms like parasites, mold, and yeast.

The wrong foods—such as sugar, processed foods, charbroiled and barbequed foods, pasta, breads, pastries, and baked goods—can increase levels of the pro-inflammatory peptides. Eat vegetables, olive and coconut oil, flax, seeds, and nuts, and take aloe vera juice.

Macular Degeneration (AMD)

This is the leading cause of blindness in people fifty-five and older. Women, drug side effects, family members who have been diagnosed with AMD, high blood pressure, smoking, and obesity have been linked to AMD. There are over ten million people in America that have this disease with a projection of millions more diagnosed by 2020. Macular degeneration occurs when the back of the eye has lost the ability to see things in detail. This makes it difficult to drive, distinguish colors or faces, or be able to read. Your sight may be strengthened by eating the Mediterranean diet, which consists of fatty fish high in omega-3, olive oil, and nuts while avoiding processed high fat foods. Eat leafy green vegetables which contain high amounts of lutein and zeaxanthin. Protect your eyes by wearing sunglasses with UVA and UVB protection and have periodic eye exams.

Osteoporosis

This disease affects over seventy-five million people who live in America, Europe, and Japan with an expectation of this figure doubling within the next fifty years. Osteoporosis is the most common bone disease leading to low bone mass and deteriorating bone structure. This disease affects more women than men and people with Asian and European ancestry. Osteoporosis increases with age. Hormonal imbalances, inflammation, high blood sugar, and significant damage to cell structures (oxidative stress) may contribute to osteoporosis. Fractures are common in the spine, hips, and forearms. You can help to maintain strong bones by eating a healthy diet of calcium sources from fruits, green leafy vegetables, beans, and yogurt. Limit red meats, caffeine, and chocolate. Do weight-bearing exercises as well as brisk walking, aerobics, and tennis. Avoid smoking, excessive drinking, and prescription drugs.

Periodontal Disease

I have a Sonicare® toothbrush. After exploring various brands on the market, I opted to go with one that had good reviews for cleaning teeth and keeping gums healthy. My mom had to have all her teeth pulled before she was fifty because the arthritis and lupus affected her circulatory system and calcium levels. I wish to keep my teeth as long as possible. Proper brushing, flossing, and regular checkups assist in stopping plaque buildup and prevent gingivitis (gum disease) from forming. Excess sugar consumption, drugs, smoking, and poor nutrition are just some of the culprits of periodontal disease. Keep your immune system healthy and eat or juice with kale, parsley, garlic, blueberry, cabbage, spinach, ginger, and pineapple. Pineapple and ginger are natural anti-inflammatories. By juicing with any of these vegetables you will be receiving the benefits of vitamin C, beta-carotene, and zinc to assist in tissue healing, strengthening the immune system, strengthening your heart, and reducing gingivitis.

Prostate

Stress and a decrease in male hormone activity may be some of the causes in prostatic hypertrophy. Add higher zinc foods like pumpkin seeds, pecans, whole grains, and lima beans. Eliminate beer, which increases prolactin, a pituitary hormone. Reducing serum cholesterol levels also helps to prevent prostate problems and inhibits tumor growth. Juice or cook with ginger, parsley, and carrots, all excellent sources of zinc. Kale and spinach elevate vitamin B6.

Shingles (Herpes Zoster)

The same virus that creates chicken pox remains in our nerve cells for years. After age fifty, one in five people will get shingles. Shingles can manifest if you are under stress, older, and have a weakened immune system. It can start as a rash on different parts of the body and then become a searing pain which can last for weeks or months depending on the severity of the attack. Help to keep your immune system elevated by eating healthy foods and removing stress from your daily life. A doctor can administer a shot which will help to fight the virus. There is no cure, however.

The Dirty Dozen

Based on 2003 United States Department of Agriculture figures, a nonprofit advocacy group, the Environmental Working Group, has listed the top twelve most contaminated fruits and vegetables.

Ranked most contaminated (in order of degree of contamination):

- Peaches
- Apples
- Bell peppers
- Celery
- Nectarines
- Strawberries
- Cherries
- Kale
- Lettuce
- Grapes (imported)
- Carrot
- Pear

Least contaminated (in order of least to most):

- Onions
- Avocados
- Sweet corn
- Pineapples
- Mangos
- Asparagus
- Sweet peas
- Kiwi
- Cabbage

- Eggplant
- Papaya
- Watermelon
- Broccoli
- Tomatoes
- Sweet Potatoes

Though I usually purchase certified organic, some non-organic produce is OK if carefully washed, as we've discussed.

Eating in Balance

The key here is creating a balance in our food intake—eating less meat and poultry, more vegetables, and less acidic protein in fish and grains. The benefits of dairy products, a source of protein, must be balanced with the drawbacks. Whey, a dairy by-product, is the basis of many protein powders. It can make your blood "dirty" while elevating the white blood cell count. Animal by-products, such as cheese, milk, and butter, can present a problem, especially if you are lactose intolerant. We believe that we must have milk and dairy in our diets to get the calcium they provide. However, an article in *Newsweek* stated that the people of Singapore consume almost no dairy and have a much lower rate of osteoporosis than the European countries that consume large amounts of dairy.

Healthy blood builds healthy flesh, bone, and muscle. We can help build our blood by consuming sixty grams of polyunsaturated fat a day, such as omega-3 and omega-6 oils, vegetable oils, seeds and nuts, flaxseed, and soybean. Greens and essential fats build healthy bodies. The plants we consume produce chlorophyll, which is vital for the body's rapid assimilation of amino acids. Its molecular structure is close to hemoglobin, which helps to increase oxygen in our system. Chlorella, a derivative from chlorophyll, is noted for improving digestion, eliminating excess mercury, balancing the body's pH, and it adds good bacteria into the intestinal tract, which helps eliminate constipation.

Re-educate yourself on a variety of healthy, nutritious foods, and eat in this new way for the rest of your life. If you consume live, healthy foods and begin and continue a sensible exercise program, your vitality will increase while you are supporting your body's many vital functions. I was recently in a store where two overweight, middle-aged women were discussing how they loved to eat their sweets and why should they deprive themselves of this pleasure? Ask yourself, "Would I rather eat healthy and live healthy for the rest of my life or overindulge and be sick for the rest of my life?" As my grandmother said, "When you have your health, you have everything." The choice is yours.

Step 4

Supplements: When (Good) Food Is Not Enough

My Story

I gradually began to take vitamin and mineral supplements in my thirties and became more of an advocate for supplements into my forties. My hormones were changing and the daily demands of being a mother of five children, and a working woman, required more support for my body. Throughout the years I have continually researched new products to assist along my path to wholeness and wellness. For a number of reasons, I find it vital to add supplements to my daily routine. Upon rising I take the following.

Ashwagandha (Winter Cherry) 570 mg

This is one of the world's most powerful adaptogens, used traditionally in Ayurvedic herbalism to help the body adapt to physiological and psychological stress. It relaxes the mind, rejuvenates the body, and increases resistance to stress.

Mitochondrial

Bodies contain organelles (little organs), which are contained in our cells. This is called mitochondria. This is our powerhouse, which supplies energy to our cells which then provide us with physical strength and stamina. As we age, our mitochondria decline, which can produce fatigue, cognitive brain malfunction, Parkinson's, and diabetes. There are several supplements available. Currently, I take a product called Mitochondrial Energy Optimizer with BioPQQ (lifeextension.org), which contains enhancing components: carnosine (antioxidant), L-Taurine (amino acid-building block of protein), benfotiamine (antioxidant), R-lipoic acid (antioxidant), BioPQQ (antioxidant).

The Gulf War veterans (1990-1991) suffered what is called "Gulf War Syndrome." Researchers at UC San Diego School of Medicine have determined that the symptoms show that the veterans have impaired functions of mitochondria, which are the powerhouse energy in cells. This 2014 discovery can assist in helping veterans become healthier as well as promote preventive measures for future veterans. Mitochondrial illnesses include muscle and exercise intolerance, fatigue, and gastrointestinal and cognitive challenges. Imaging technology was used to compare veterans with Gulf War illness to healthy veterans. The study consisted of fourteen people—seven with illnesses from the war and seven matching controls. Age, ethnicity, and sex were considered. The technique used—31-phosphorus magnetic resonance spectroscopy or 31P-MRS—reveals amounts of phosphorus-containing compounds in cells. Such compounds are important for cell energy production, in particular phosphocreatine or PCr, which declines in muscle cells during exercise. The principal investigator was Beatrice A. Golomb MD, PhD, professor of medicine along with associate Hayley Koslik and Gavin Hamilton, PhD, a research scientist and magnetic resonance physicist. They used the imaging technology to compare Gulf War veterans with diagnosed Gulf War illness to healthy controls. "Some have sought to ascribe Gulf War illness to stress," said Golomb "Gulf War illness was also contributed to nerve gas and nerve gas pre-treatment pills given to troops. Patients with mitochondrial dysfunction were also similar to Gulf War patients. These inhibitors have known mitochondrial toxicity and generally show the strongest and most consistent relationship to predicting Gulf War illness. Mitochondrial problems account for which exposures relate to Gulf War illness, which symptoms predominate, how Gulf War illness symptoms manifest themselves, what objective tests have been altered, and why routine blood tests have not been useful" (2014).

Suggested Reading

Aubrey DeGrey's *Mitochondrial Free Radical Theory of Aging 14 and Reductive Hotspot Hypothesis of Aging.*

I also take a digestive enzyme with cooked foods. At bedtime, I drink a magnesium and calcium drink along with a capsule of melatonin for sound sleep. When I travel, I carry labeled vitamin boxes.

This is my current program. Everyone has their own personal needs depending on age, health, and activity. I highly suggest you tap into your own personal supplement support. I am a bargain shopper and have researched where to buy quality supplements that offer deeper discounts.

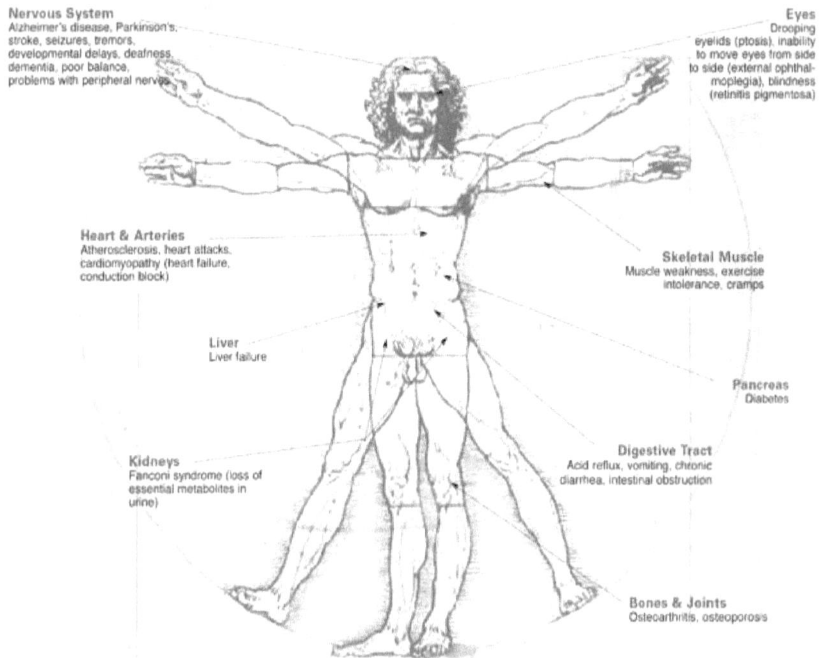

Host Defense

Paul Stamets, founder of Host Defense Mushrooms, is a mycologist and author of six books on mushroom cultivation and identification, including the definitive text *Growing Gourmet & Medicinal Mushrooms*. The Washington State Department of Agriculture as well as being gluten-free, non-GMO, and bee friendly certify his mushroom products as organic. Host Defense carries a multitude of mushroom products that assist in helping the body: heart, immune, stress, respiratory, oxygen, free radical damage, kidney, energy, stamina, mental clarity, cerebral and mental support, normalizing blood sugar, digestive, lymphatic, hormones and adrenals, liver, and brain.

Spring and Fall Detox

No matter how clean our diet is or how we reduce stress in our daily lives, the use of drugs, toxins in our environment and traveling contribute to the overall decline of our health. Detoxing is great for our bodies if done twice yearly in spring and fall. Some of the symptoms that let us know our bodies are toxic are:

- Constipation
- Excessive diarrhea
- Chronic fatigue
- Joint and muscle pain
- Insomnia
- Bloating
- Increased belly fat

Optimoxx is a product that has two individual formulas. One works on the colon and lymphatic system. The second formula works on liver and kidney support.

Supplements and Health: The Benefits

With today's agriculture methods, we can no longer be sure we are receiving the nutrients necessary for our optimum health. Our soil is often depleted, mass food production is not always of the best quality and genetically modified foods (GMOs) are becoming more and more prevalent in the food industry. Our diets are just not as wholesome as they were in our grandparents' day. Though they may have consumed large quantities of dairy, meat, eggs, and other foods that were home grown or produced by their neighbors, those foods contained few food additives and preservatives which today are "required" to preserve freshness or color.

If you eat a moderate amount of fast or processed foods and also have a high level of stress in your life, you definitely will want to consider consulting with your physician/naturopath about adding supplements to your diet.

Synthetic Supplements

- Laboratory conditions may block the production of natural vitamins.
- May contain food dyes which can block absorption of B complex vitamins.
- Do not contain high levels of antioxidants.
- May be made under high heat conditions which over time can produce toxins into the body.

Natural Food Base Supplements

- Provide a full complement of fruits and vegetables which the normal person doesn't consume on a daily basis.
- They do not contain chemicals.
- Since these are food-based, do your homework on various companies to research the quality of the food source.
- Remember to educate yourself on supplement ingredients.

Daily Supplements: The Basics

Multivitamin/Mineral Complex

Functions and Uses

Many people take a multivitamin/mineral complex every day. They commonly contain thirteen of the essential vitamins, the complete

B complex, and vital minerals. There are multi-supplements that are geared for pregnant women, men and women over fifty, and people whose poor nutritional habits need assistance and more nourishment in receiving certain nutrients. Minerals help our cells grow and stay healthy as well as working in synergy with other minerals and vitamins to support vital body functions.

Dosages

Dosages may vary depending on the measurement of ingredients. The recommended dietary allowance (RDA) does not always support certain needs, thus higher strengths may be necessary.

Health Benefits

Vegetarians, as well as people who participate in excessive exercise or experience high stress, benefit by receiving more nutrients. If you eat a consistent diet of cooked and processed foods, you can also benefit by taking a daily supplement. If you do not take supplements, you can receive multiple benefits by taking an all-around supplement; however, be sure you select one of high quality.

Vitamin B Complex

There are eight components that make up this water-soluble complex, each having its own specialized functions for the body. One can take a B complex which would include the following components:

Water-Soluble Vitamins
Water-soluble means that the pill dissolves in water and is not stored in the liver or fat.

B-1 Thiamine

Functions and Uses

Thiamine supports the heart, muscles, and nervous system and helps to convert carbohydrates into energy. People who are thiamine deficient can experience leg cramps, muscle weakness, and swelling of the heart. A recent study by the researchers at the

University of Warwick in the UK has revealed that high doses of vitamin B1 or thiamine can also reverse early diabetic kidney disease. Diabetes is the most frequent cause of kidney failure, accounting for nearly 45 percent of new cases in America alone. Patients with type 2 diabetes, once known as non-insulin-dependent diabetes or adult-onset diabetes, are at much greater risk of developing kidney disease. The onset of kidney disease can be evaluated by a high excretion rate of the protein albumin from the body in the urine through the process known as microalbuminuria; the study at the University of Warwick confirmed that patients taking thiamine for three months showed marked lessening of albumin in the urine.

Dosage

A normal dose is 1.8 mg to 3 mg. Larger amounts have been known to cause toxicity.

B-1 Health Benefits

- Better digestion.
- Improved mental ability.
- Aids in reducing stress and depression.
- Thiamine is found in wheat germ, eggs, leafy green vegetables, legumes, nuts, and enriched cereals.

B-2 Riboflavin

Functions and Uses

It requires the body to use oxygen and metabolize fatty acids, carbohydrates, and amino acids. Deficiencies may show up as sores around the mouth, inflamed tongue, eye disorders, light sensitivity, dizziness, hair lose, and insomnia.

Dosage

The average dosage is 50 mg per day along with 50 mg of B-6. For better absorption, take with vitamin C. Higher amounts can be taken if on a weight loss diet, under stress, drinking alcohol, or taking antibiotics.

B-2 Health Benefits

- Healthier skin, hair, and nails.
- Increases energy in the body.
- Supports healthy red blood cells.
- Provides antioxidants to help slow down aging.
- Foods that are high in B-2 are yogurt, fish, green leafy vegetables, dairy, nuts, and grains.

B-3 Niacin—Nicotinic Acid—Vitamin P or Vitamin PP

Functions and Uses

It is found in plants and animal tissues. In 1915, Dr. Joseph Goldberger discovered a link between prison inmates fed low amounts of niacin through their diet. He coined the word "pellagra" (the disease of the four Ds: dementia, diarrhea, dermatitis, and death). By adding niacin rich foods Dr. Goldberg was able to reverse the inmates' symptoms.

Dosage

The suggested RDA is 19 mg for males and 13 mg for females per day. Too little produces mental confusion, irritability, and diarrhea. Alcoholism can make people deficient in B-3. Harmless flushing of the skin may occur, but if a medical condition arises, it is advisable to consult with your practitioner about taking higher dosages.

B-3 Health Benefits

- Supports the nervous system, sex hormones, skin, stomach, intestinal tract, and removes toxins.
- Reduces bad cholesterol (LDL) and increases good cholesterol (HDL) and promotes better circulation.

- Helps with osteoarthritis, rheumatoid arthritis, and insulin-dependent diabetes.
- Food sources include salmon, tuna, chicken, peas, dried beans, sunflower seeds, beets, brewer's yeast, veal, pork, and turkey.

B Vitamin Rich Foods

Foods that have B vitamin benefits include green vegetables, whole grains, lentils, potatoes, bananas, dairy products, eggs, turkey liver, and tuna. Take B complex earlier in the day. Taking B complex later may interrupt a sound sleep.

Pantothenic Acid B-5

Functions and Uses

B-5 plays a role in metabolizing fats, carbohydrates, and proteins. Pantothenic acid is an essential nutrient to sustain life. People take B-5 for dietary deficiencies, to lower blood sugar, and to treat respiratory disorders, carpal tunnel syndrome, depression, fatigue, celiac disease, headaches, asthma, osteo- and rheumatoid arthritis, Parkinson's disease, shingles, enlarged prostate, and multiple sclerosis. It also helps produce vitamin D.

Dosage

The average dosage is 5 mg although people may take up to 250 mg a day. Too much pantothenic acid can produce anxiety and overstimulation and may lead to diarrhea.

B-5 Health Benefits

- More vitality
- Better moods
- Alertness
- Wound healing
- Food sources include yogurt, avocados, peas, beans,

poultry, and organ meats

B-6 Pyridoxine

The blood and nervous system require B-6 to function well. It converts tryptophan (amino acid) to niacin. B-6 makes hemoglobin, which carries oxygen to tissues. B-6 deficiency can make one iron deficient and anemic. Other symptoms caused by B-6 deficiency include dermatitis, confusion, and depression.

Dosage

The RDA recommendation for people over age fifty is 1.5 mg for women, 1.7 mg for men. For adults, it is considered safe to take from 50 to 100 mg per day. When taken in high doses (200 mg or more per day) over a long period of time, vitamin B-6 can cause neurological disorders such as loss of sensation in legs and imbalance. Symptoms are reversed when that dosage is no longer taken.

B-6 Health Benefits

- Balances estrogen and progesterone levels.
- Acts as a diuretic.
- Formation of red blood cells.
- Regulates blood pressure.
- Improves the nervous system.
- Food sources high in B-6 include calves' liver, sardines, snapper, shrimp, halibut, Chinook salmon, lamb, beef tenderloin, and venison.

Vitamin B-12 Cobalamin

Functions and Uses

This is the most complex of the B vitamins. A vegetarian diet is more likely to be deficient in B-12 than one which includes meat, fish, eggs, and milk.

Deficiencies in B-12 may also be caused by malabsorption, which can lead to pernicious anemia. Pernicious anemia destroys intrinsic factor (IF), an enzyme secreted by the stomach and necessary to produce B-12. B-12 deficiency may cause dementia, which is closely correlated to the early stages of Alzheimer's disease. Lower levels of B-12 may elevate homocysteine (amino acid), which may lead to heart disease. Depression, memory problems, and nervousness also may be signs of a deficiency. Taking B-12 in conjunction with folic acid and B complex helps improve healthy heart functions.

Dosage

Absorption of B-12 can decrease with age. B-12 is stored in small amounts in the body, so daily doses may not be required. The RDA for adults is currently 2.4 mcg per day but can range as high as 3,000 mcg daily. According to the Institute of Medicine of the National Academy of Sciences, there are no adverse effects from large doses of vitamin B-12. People with eating disorders, inflammatory stomach, and intestinal disorders may require higher dosages, as their ingestion of B-12 can be slowed. B-12 also can be absorbed through a skin patch, injection, or sublingual tablet. If you question your B-12 levels, there are numerous tests to evaluate whether you are low in this B vitamin. It is impossible for the body to store too much B-12.

B-12 Health Benefits

- Healthy nervous system
- Better digestion
- Carbohydrate metabolism
- More energy
- Sharper memory
- Fewer migraines
- Improved skin, nails, and hair

- Food sources high in B-12 include shellfish, lamb and beef liver, mackerel, herring, salmon, tuna, beef, cheese, and eggs

Folic Acid—Folate—Folinic Acid

Functions and Uses

Folic acid manufactures red blood cells and a lack of it may cause anemia. It lowers homocysteine (amino acid) levels to help improve heart health. High levels of homocysteine have been connected to Alzheimer's disease, strokes, and osteoporosis. Low levels of folic acid have been linked to alcoholism, liver disease, and colon and cervical cancer. Pregnant women need to take folic acid to prevent spina bifida (spine and back misdevelopment) in the fetus. People who are on kidney dialysis can also benefit by taking folic acid.

Dosage

A normal dose is 400 mcg per day. During the early stages of pregnancy, the recommended dosage is 400 to 800 mcg per day. If you have health issues, consult with your practitioner regarding how much folic acid you should take.

Folic Acid Health Benefits

- Strengthens fragile bones (osteoporosis).
- Lifts depression.
- Helps improve macular degeneration (eye disease).
- Wards off hearing loss.
- Improves memory.
- Deters Alzheimer's disease.

B-7 Biotin—Vitamin H

Functions and Uses

Biotin research began in the early 1900s. The research went on for forty years before it was acknowledged as a vitamin. Biotin is important in cell growth as well as metabolizing fats and amino acids. It helps the body to use glucose (blood sugar) for body fluids. Deficiencies include hair loss, rash around the mouth, eyes and nose, tingling in the arms and legs, depression, brittle nails and thinning hair. Biotin has been coined the "beauty vitamin" and is included in many hair and nail products.

Dosage

The suggested dosage is 30 to 100 mcg daily. Higher amounts up to 2,500 mcg have been safe to take. Diabetics have taken 5 to 1.5 mg to help reduce their blood sugar.

B-7 Health Benefits

- Strengthens hair and nails.
- Good for weight loss.
- Biotin combined with chromium may help reduce blood sugar in diabetics.
- Foods which contain biotin are egg yolks, brewer's yeast, wheat germ, molasses, peanuts and peanut butter, oatmeal, beans and legumes, fish, breads, poultry, cauliflower, mushrooms, dairy products, and bananas.

B Vitamin Dosages

Before taking a B complex supplement, you might want to consult your health-care provider. People's bodies vary, and while some may require a higher dosage of B-12, for example, others would benefit from a higher ratio of another of the B vitamins.

Vitamin C—Ascorbic Acid

Functions and Uses

This supplement is a water-soluble antioxidant nutrient which helps block free radicals from building up which create aging in the body. Deficiencies in vitamin C can cause bleeding gums, bruising, decrease in the body's ability to fight infections, painful and swollen joints, and rough skin.

Linus Pauling was a renowned scientist and winner of the Nobel Peace Prize. This remarkable man was a strong advocate for taking increasingly higher dosages of vitamin C to ward off diseases and the common cold. He coined the term "orthomolecular," meaning the right molecules in the right amount. His research on vitamin C has been highly debated throughout the years. He died at the age of 94.

Dosage

Suggested dose is 2,000 mg daily or lower. Some side effects of higher amounts may include diarrhea and stomach upset. Vitamin C comes in powder and pill variety. I prefer the powder added to water, juice, or into a protein drink.

Vitamin C Health Benefits

- Helps heal wounds.
- Builds stronger bones, cartilage, and teeth.
- As an antioxidant, vitamin C helps fight off diseases like cancer, heart disease, and inflammatory conditions such as arthritis.

Foods High in Vitamin C

Food sources of vitamin C are broccoli, brussels sprouts, cabbage, cauliflower, red peppers, winter squash, leafy greens, raspberries, cranberries, blueberries, and pineapple.

Vitamin D

Functions and Uses

As children we were told to drink our milk for our bone health because that, along with diet, would supply our daily dose of vitamin D. Medical doctors are now recognizing that vitamin D is playing biologic roles in peoples' health, thanks to Dr. Michael Holick, the world's leading researcher on vitamin D. According to his research, vitamin D appears to play a vital role in cancer prevention as well as cancer treatment. Deficiencies show up as aches, pains, and weakness in muscles and bones. Many people are vitamin D deficient compared to our hunter ancestors who were exposed to the sun all day. Because of the rise in skin cancer, it is now recommended that we wear sunscreen protection and do not expose ourselves to the sun between 10:00 a.m. and 2:00 p.m. However, our bodies only produce vitamin D during those hours. The cold winter months contribute to vitamin D deficiency as well. If we are not to be in the sun as our ancestors were, we may need to consider supplementation.

Dosage

Dr. Holick suggests that children need a daily dose of between 400 and 1,000 IU; teenagers and adults between 1,500 and 2,000 IU daily. Since older people produce 75 percent less vitamin D in the body, Dr. Holick recommends that people over the age of seventy have more sun exposure to their backs, legs, arms, and abdomen while protecting their face. According to a study done in 2003 with Dr. Robert Heaney of Creighton University Research Center, one can take 10,000 IU of vitamin D daily for six months without toxicity. One can take D with or without food daily, weekly, or monthly as long as you receive the recommended dose.

Vitamin D Health Benefits

- Improves mood.
- Helps build bone mass.
- Prevents autoimmune disease, colds, and flu.

- May also help to reduce risks of cancer, decrease inflammation and chronic pain.
- Helps obese people by stimulating fat cell metabolism.
- Stimulates insulin production for diabetics.
- Good food sources include dairy products, wild caught salmon, sardines, shrimp, halibut, trout, tofu, soy milk, milk, and orange juice.

Vitamin E—D-Alpha-Tocopherol

Functions and Uses

This is a fat-soluble vitamin which can be stored in the body up to six months. It comes in eight different forms with d-alpha-tocopherol being the most active. It also acts as a powerful antioxidant which protects cells against free radicals, therefore helping to protect the body from cancer and cardiovascular diseases that can occur when cells are damaged. Gamma-tocopherol is less strong but very essential for maintaining healthy cell membranes, especially when d-alpha-tocopherol is present. A recent study done by Australia's Queensland University of Technology demonstrates that gamma-tocopherol has the ability to inhibit prostate cancer stem cells.

Dosage

The recommended amount is 800 to 1,600 mg per day, if not consuming vitamin E from food sources. Otherwise, absorption of vitamin A and K can be compromised. Other forms of vitamin E can be taken. The cold-water form (alpha tocopherol succinate/acetate) is twice as expensive as the soy-based oil. It is effectively absorbed on an empty stomach if taken with several grams of a fat or oil. A second form is soybean oil (E-acetate), which is low in saturated fat and does not contain cholesterol. Liquid vitamin E absorbs better than the capsule form. Selenium, magnesium, and vitamin A will increase the benefits of vitamin E.

Vitamin E Health Benefits

- Reduces cholesterol; lowers chances of stroke and coronary artery disease.
- Helps protect eyes.
- Protects against UV radiation.
- Heals wounds.
- Keeps skin moist.
- Helps relieve arthritic pain.
- Good food sources include wheat germ oil, almonds, sunflower seeds, mustard and turnip greens, and spinach.

Vitamin K

Functions and Uses

This fat-soluble supplement was discovered by Edward Adelbert Doisy and Henrik Dam who won a Nobel Peace Prize in 1943. The "K" stands for the German word *koagulation*, as it assists in coagulating blood. It also assists in normal bone calcification. Low vitamin K is associated with lower bone density and common hip fractures and often can affect the elderly. Deficiencies show up as bruising and bleeding. People on antibiotics show poor absorption of K in the intestinal tract.

Dosage

If you are on an anticoagulant drug, consult with your physician before taking vitamin K. Consider obtaining a supplement that contains all three of the K forms: MK-7, MK-4, and K1. Although a small amount of K (80mcg) is sufficient for clotting blood, higher dosages are beneficial for age-related diseases and safe to take.

Vitamin K Health Benefits

- Fewer heart attacks.

- Increases bone mass in post-menopausal women.
- Regulates blood sugar.
- Reduces bone fractures, especially in post-menopausal women.
- Treats heavy menstrual bleeding.
- Promotes normal blood clotting.
- Good food sources include brussels sprouts, spinach, kale, cauliflower, broccoli, cabbage, and soybeans.

Good to Consider Supplements

Calcium (CA) Calcium Carbonate—Calcium Citrate—Calcium Malate

Functions and Uses

This major mineral is primarily stored in the bones and teeth with smaller amounts found in the blood, muscles, and extra cellular fluid. At a younger age, the body continues to break calcium down and build it up to help support strong bones. As we age, calcium requirements become higher because the mineral becomes stored in the body more than it's replenished.

Dosage

Dosages may vary depending on age. After age fifty the requirement is at 1,200 mg per day. Taking vitamin D with calcium helps to absorb the calcium into your body. If you take more than 2,500 mg per day, it may interfere with other minerals as well as affect healthy kidney functions. If you have certain health conditions such as heart problems, bone tumors, or kidney problems, consult your physician to determine whether this is a supplement you can take.

Calcium Health Benefits

- Treats osteoporosis.
- Helps to build bones.
- May help control high blood pressure.
- Protects pre-menopausal women against breast cancer.
- Calcium is found in milk, cheese, yogurt, sardines, broccoli, kale, and dark green leafy vegetables.

Magnesium (MG)

Functions and Uses

Magnesium is a crucial mineral which supports over 300 chemical reactions in the body to have it work efficiently. Our soil is depleted of MG due to the use of fertilizers. Though the normal body contains 25 grams, it is common for women, African Americans, and the elderly to have a magnesium deficiency. Surface water contains very small amounts of MG and certain medicines can also deplete magnesium in the body. Magnesium deficiency may create physical and mental stress and loss of potassium and calcium through urination.

Dosage

Many calcium and magnesium supplements have a ratio of 2:1 calcium to magnesium. For instance, if your supplement contains 1,200 mg of calcium, the magnesium would be 600 mg. If you have a kidney disease or other conditions, consult with your physician before taking.

Magnesium Health Benefits

- Assists in heart regulation.
- Promotes healthy bones.
- Normal blood pressure.

- Helps treat diabetes.
- Treats kidney stones.
- Relieves asthma.
- Helps people with multiple sclerosis.
- Reduces migraine headaches.
- Helps altitude sickness.
- Helps stomach acid.

Foods High in Magnesium

Some foods that contain magnesium are broccoli, squash, dark green leafy vegetables, beans, whole grains, chocolate, coffee, and almonds.

Coenzyme Q10—CoQ10

Functions and Uses

This fat-soluble vitamin-like compound called ubiquinone plays an important role inside our human cells, allowing for healthy cellular growth, energy production, and immune and antioxidant support. The highest amount of CoQ10 is found in the heart. There have been numerous scientific studies done on the benefits of taking CoQ10. Many have to do with heart disease. Unusually low levels of CoQ10 have been reported with people who have high blood pressure.

Dosage

A healthy adult can take between 30 and 100 mg per day. People who have heart conditions may take dosages of 150 mg per day with a practitioner's consultation. Some studies have linked the diminishing of women's breast tumors after taking 390 mg for one month. CoQ10 assimilates best when taken with a small amount of fat such as peanut butter or olive oil.

CoQ10 Health Benefits

- Prevents fatty acid buildup within the heart muscle.
- Converts to energy, which assists the heart in functioning better.
- Helps with high blood pressure.
- Helps chronic fatigue.
- Aids in weight loss.

Essential Fatty Acids—EFAs

Functions and Uses

EFAs are found in every cell throughout our body. Omega-3 ALA (alpha linoleic acid) is vital because of its ability to suppress inflammation in the body, which helps prevent degenerative diseases such as heart disease, Alzheimer's, rheumatoid arthritis, and diabetes. Eight percent of the brain's weight consists of omega-3s. This contributes to improved memory, mental health, and Alzheimer's prevention. People who are depressed or have attempted or committed suicide have been shown to have reduced levels of DHA and EPA in their red blood cell membranes or serum. Unlike omega-3, omega-6 creates inflammation. The healthy ratio between omega-6 and omega-3 is a range of 3:1 (3 parts omega-3 to 1 part omega-6) or 4:1 (4 parts omega-3 to 1 part omega-6).

Dosage

Omega-3s 1,000 to 3,000 mg of EFA and 1,000 to 1,500 mg of DHA. One need not take omega-6 in pill form if omega-6 food sources are consumed on a daily basis or a pharmaceutical grade of EFAs oil contains a ratio of 3:1 or 4:1.

EFAs/Omega-3 Health Benefits

- Anti-inflammatory.
- Relieves menopause symptoms.

- Alleviates depression.
- Helps heart, breast, and bone health.
- Reduces high blood pressure.
- Relieves arthritis symptoms.
- Reduces high cholesterol.
- Reverses early stages of Alzheimer's.
- Helps prevent osteoporosis.
- Helps prevent obesity.
- Helps prevent prostate problems.
- Omega-3 food sources include wild salmon, sardines, herring, mackerel, flaxseed, walnuts, pumpkin seeds, eggs, fruits, vegetables, and olive oil.

Omega-6 Health Benefits

- Maintains healthy brain function.
- Reduces nerve pain for diabetic neuropathy.
- Reduces pain and swelling for rheumatoid arthritic conditions.
- Builds strong bones.
- Promotes healthy skin.
- Helps alleviate hot flashes and night sweats.
- Omega-6 food sources are evening primrose oil, borage oil, sunflower oil, olive oil, safflower oil, wheat germ oil, flaxseed oil, sesame oil, hempseed oil, almonds, pistachios, olives, chicken, and turkey.

Conjugated Linoleic Acid (CLA)

Functions and Uses

Approximately 34 percent of the current US population is classified as obese.

One billion people worldwide are obese according to the World Health Organization (WHO). Weight escalates during holiday seasons when we all tend to overeat. If CLA can contribute to reducing body fat and slowing or reversing weight gain (according to the *International Journal of Obesity* and Professor Schoeller), then doesn't it make sense to take CLA along with your sensible nutrition and exercise plan?

CLA helps the body break down and use the fat normally stored after meals. It decreases body fat mass, maintains lean body mass, and aids in weight management—reducing the "yo-yo" effect often associated with diet plans. A study published in late 2005 by the Journal of Nutrition found that adults taking a CLA supplement lost as much as 9 percent of their body fat. As important, a follow-up, twelve-month study found that participants did not regain their body fat.

To get three grams of CLA through food alone, an adult would have to consume more than four gallons of ice cream or twenty-eight quarter-pound hamburgers every day. Obviously, CLA supplementation is the only way to go. Supplementation with CLA is most effective as part of a daily regimen that includes exercise and a reasonable diet.

Dosage

With each meal, take 1,000 mg of CLA. Tonalin® CLA is derived from natural safflower oil and the company claims it is the most clinically tested CLA on the market. Tonalin® CLA is stimulant-free and is available in health food stores, retail chains, and online.

CLA Health Benefits

- Reduces body fat.

- Increases cholesterol metabolism.
- Lowers triglycerides.
- Lowers insulin resistance.
- Enhances immune system.

Lutein

Functions and Uses

This is a naturally occurring carotenoid which is a natural coloring found in vegetables and fruits. This supplement plays a critical role in support of healthy eyes. It acts as a protection from blue light in indoor lighting as well as sunlight.

Dosage

Take 6 to 10 mg of lutein and 1 mg of zeaxanthin daily. For older people with poor digestion, a sublingual spray is available.

Lutein Health Benefits

- May help reduce cataracts.
- May help reduce risks of age-related macular degeneration (AMD).
- May supply antioxidant properties.
- Lutein is naturally found in foods which include dark green leafy vegetables, romaine lettuce, pistachio nuts, and egg yolks.

Chromium

This is an essential trace mineral which helps to regulate sugar through the cells and reduce glucose levels in the blood. People with type 1 and type 2 mellitus diabetes may benefit by taking this supplement. Consult with your physician.

Dosage

A suggested dosage is between 50 and 200 mg daily. The side effects are rare at these dosages.

Chromium Health Benefits

- May help control abnormal glucose intolerance in type 2 diabetes.
- May help to control cholesterol levels.
- May help to control fat.
- May help reduce cravings for sweets.
- Food sources include eggs, brewer's yeast, chicken, potatoes, apples, peas, broccoli, and mushrooms.

Alpha-Lipoic Acid

This sulfur-containing fatty acid is present in all human cells. In 1988, alpha-lipoic acid was recognized as an effective antioxidant which helps to neutralize free radicals that can damage cells. Free radicals contribute to aging and chronic illnesses. It also increases the production of glutathione which helps to dissolve toxic substances from the liver. It may help people with cataracts, glaucoma, multiple sclerosis, Parkinson's, and Alzheimer's disease.

Dosage

If you are healthy, dosages are 50 to 300 mg daily. For people who have diabetes, 100 to 200 mg three times a day is a suggested dosage. Taking dosages higher than 1,800 mg could cause headaches, nausea, and low blood sugar.

Alpha-Lipoic Health Benefits

- May help the body utilize insulin more effectively.
- May help with inflammation in joints, arteries, and muscles.

- Improves blood flow and circulation to the body and the brain.
- Helps to reduce environmental toxins to the cells.
- Helps strengthen heart muscles and arteries.
- Food sources include peas, broccoli, brussels sprouts, and spinach.

Store supplements in a cupboard away from heat and check expiration dates on bottles. Some supplements require refrigeration after opening. Educate yourself on brands with a good reputation and look to see if they are synthetic or natural. If in doubt, consult with a physician, naturopath, health food expert or other professional familiar with this topic. If you are under a physician's care for a chronic health problem, consult with your doctor before taking any supplements.

Supplements, Drug Therapies, and Health Conditions

Insomnia

Each person has their own definition of insomnia. 30 to 50 percent of people have acknowledged having occasional insomnia while 10 percent are chronic insomniacs. It appears that women are more affected than men. Aging, excessive drinking, stress, depression, and poor mental health can all play a role in our sleeping patterns. Physiological causes range from circadian rhythm disorders to a host of physical conditions including chronic pain, heart problems, sleep apnea, asthma, Parkinson's disease, Alzheimer's disease, and disturbances of the brain such as strokes and brain tumors.

Hormones and Sleep

Our bodies normally produce human growth hormone (HGH), which aids in sleep. Our adrenal glands are restored during sleep; but with lack of sleep, cortisol, which is produced through our adrenals, becomes elevated and results in sluggishness, constipation, PMS, bloating, and a low libido. By the time we reach fifty, the amount of sleep we get begins to decline by 27 percent a decade, and HGH secretion decreases by 78 percent over this period. Less HGH is produced by the body because of less deep sleep. However, HGH replacement therapy has confirmed that patients taking HGH sleep better.

Excess fat in the body can destroy HGH levels.

Supplement Suggestions before Bedtime

- Melatonin
- Valerian
- DHEA
- Calcium—magnesium
- Chamomile tea
- Tryptophan
- 5-HTP

Depression

Over fourteen million Americans have been diagnosed with depression. There are a multitude of causes. It could be a loss of a loved one, a loss of a job or home, health conditions, being older or shifts in hormones and medications. Depressed people seem to lose interest in life, become anxious or irritable, and may even contemplate suicide.

Supplement Suggestions

- Omega-3 fatty acids
- SAM-e
- Folic acid

- Magnesium
- Tryptophan
- Morpheme Memocare (Ayurvedic)
- Licorice tea
- St. John's Wort

Osteoporosis

When my mother slipped in the tub and broke her hip, she had been on steroid medication for an accelerated rheumatoid arthritic condition, and the steroid treatments were not supplemented with any vitamins or minerals. Statistically, there is a 30 percent mortality rate within the first year after suffering a hip fracture. My mother lived for seven more years, but not without constant pain, swelling, and an ambulatory condition which severely compromised her health. She developed lupus and had a stroke in her early fifties.

Osteoporosis causes a loss of bone density, contributing to the one and a half million fractures (including 300,000 broken hips) suffered annually. Women especially face bone loss during menopause due to reduced estrogen production. Contrary to popular belief, men can also be affected by osteoporosis, but usually five to ten years after women.

My family history showed no indication of RA. Observing and living with a parent who experienced constant severe pain was emotionally difficult for family members; however, her condition helped me to become more aware of my own well-being and thus I became more health minded through my lifetime.

Supplement Suggestions

- Calcium, vitamin D, zinc, copper, magnesium, boron.
- Vitamin C, B12, vitamin K, folic acid, and silicon are essential for stronger bones.

- Trace minerals and magnesium can help support healthy bone function.
- Take 1,000 IU of vitamin D, 1,200 milligrams of calcium and 400 milligrams of magnesium.

If you wish to research this subject further, refer to the references at the end of the book. This offers a wealth of research as well as advice on supplements and diagnostic testing. In chapter three, the Healthy Numbers section also provides more information on osteoporosis.

When to Take Supplements

A suggestion is to take amino acids on an empty stomach. For better absorption take fat-soluble supplements with foods that contains oil or fat. Take supplements at breakfast and lunch. Herbal sleep aids can be taken an hour before bedtime.

Menopause

My Menopause Story

While in my upper forties, I began to experience pre-menopausal symptoms which included night sweats, irregular menstrual cycles, poor sleeping patterns, and emotional irritations. It wasn't until I almost reached fifty that I was post-menopausal. I was and still remain very physical. I read once that a professional ballet dancer can exhibit irregular hormones and experience cessation of her menstrual cycle at a young age due to vigorous training, but once she stops her training, her cycle returns to normal. I began my cycle when I was twelve years old, so I reasoned that I was approaching post-menopause at an earlier age. I had never gone on birth control, nor was I a pharmaceutical or over-the-counter user, so I visited my doctor of Chinese medicine. The doctor prescribed Chinese medicine and gave me a series of acupuncture treatments that helped to lessen some of the symptoms, and I rode it out. There weren't any bio-identical testing methods back then and because my preference had always been to go the herbal route, that felt like the best course for me to take.

Hormone Replacement Therapy

Wyeth Pharmaceuticals, manufacturers of Premarin® and Prempro® is asking the FDA to deny Americans access to bio-identical hormone replacement drugs prepared by compounding pharmacies and available only under a doctor's prescription. These custom-made preparations combine individualized doses of hormones chemically identical to those found in the human body. Prescription hormones such as Premarin® are proving to have certain unsafe side effects, leading to more physicians prescribing bio-identical hormone replacement therapies.

Bio-identical formulations can be made without the additives and dyes commonly found in conventional, one-size-fits-all prescription drugs. Moreover, the use of compounded hormones allows for specialized, flexible dosing strategies. This is consistent with the most recent FDA Menopause and Fact Sheet (issued in July 2005), which recommends that menopausal hormone therapy should be used at the lowest doses for the shortest duration needed to achieve treatment goals. Hormones decrease dramatically in aging adults, including menopausal women. Lowered hormone production associated with age results in decreased bone mass, hot flashes, diminished libido, vaginal dryness, allergies, fatigue, poor sleep, sugar cravings, excess fat, and memory lapses.

Restoring hormones for men and women alike will produce many benefits including relief from depression, insomnia, migraine headaches, low energy, low libido, and mental fatigue.

Get advice from your physician or health-care practitioner before starting hormone replacement therapy during and after menopause.

Hormone/Insulin-Cortisol Balance

Refined sugar and starchy foods create an overload of blood sugar and when it hits our cells, blood sugar levels drop. Decreased blood sugar levels create stress in our brains and cortisol kicks in. Stress produces higher levels of cortisol, which in turn depletes progesterone levels. Our bodies use progesterone as a building block to make cortisol, so when we manufacture high levels of cortisol, we deplete progesterone and disrupt its balance with estrogen.

Insulin is a hormone that transports blood sugar to our cells to be used as energy. When our body is producing excess amounts of cortisol, overweight individuals can become insulin-resistant, becoming more immune to insulin's effects.

Supplement Suggestions

- Soy isoflavones—40 mg daily.
- Indole-3-carbinol—300-500 mg daily.
- Chromium—200-600 mg daily.
- DHEA—10-25 mg daily; monitor reaction.
- L-carnitine—500 mg daily.
- CoQ10—100-200 mg daily.
- Red clover (trifolium pratense)—helps with hot flashes, contains high levels of isoflavones (estrogen-like plant compounds). 15 to 30 drops, three times daily; do not use with blood-thinning drugs; helps improve cardiovascular health.
- Vitex/chasteberry (vitex agnus-castus)—30 drops or one cup of tea three times daily; results may be felt after three months; helps regulate progesterone and estrogen levels; calms anxiety, bloating, irritability, and depression.
- Black cohosh (cimicifuga racemosa)—40 mg daily. Contraindications: headache, nausea; is an alternative to hormone replacement therapy; helps relieve hot flashes, mood swings, and vaginal dryness; improves bone strength;

and most importantly, doesn't raise estrogen levels.

- B complex—50-100 mg daily.
- Vitamin C/bioflavonoids—1,000-2,000 mg daily.
- Calcium—1,200 mg daily.
- Magnesium glycinate—400 mg daily.
- Magnesium oxide—600 mg. (Rule of thumb: magnesium dosage is usually one-half of calcium dosage, i.e., 1,200 mg calcium=600 mg of magnesium).
- Fish oil—5,000 mg daily.
- Zinc—25-50 mg daily.

Alzheimer's

Alzheimer's is the third leading cause of death in the U.S. This disease is related to anything inflammatory, such as leaky gut, pathogens, toxicity, energy, and anything low in trophic side: nerve growth factors, BDNF (brain derived neurotrophic factor) related to memory and learning, estradiol (estrogen steroid hormone), nutrients, Vitamin D.

Causes include sleep apnea, vascular occlusion, pathogens, and sinusitis.

For optimal brain health, we need good blood flow, exercise, oxygenation, mitochondrial function, and metabolic flexibility. This is similar to what can cause Parkinsons, ALS, and macular degeneration—insufficiency in a subsystem with brains undersupported. This is why it may be important to collaborate with a neurologist as well as an internal physician trained in functional medicine, which is a more modern concept of diagnosis.

Alzheimer's takes twenty years to develop the disease. Preventative measures within the first ten years include a cognoscope blood test, Vitamin D, hormones, and prediabetes and toxicity testing. There are also online cognitive assessments people can take. Additional MRI testing can be done.

Data shown in JAMA (Journal of the American Medical Association) and Lancet report that certain people who were diagnosed with COVID-19 had neurological dysfunctions.

People can be aware of several symptoms regarding brain dysfunction: faster heart rate, poor sleep, and lower oxygen, as well as high stress.

Environmental hazards have played a part in brain dysfunctions. The 9/11 tragedy affected many firefighters and rescuers with toxins that were diagnosed as late as 2015. The massive California fires also impacted health.

Glyphosate is an agricultural herbicide that pollutes rivers, streams, and water sources and creates toxicity, which may also affect the brain. We do not live in a pristine environment.

Preventative measures to be taken before the disease can no longer be treated would include, first, removing the health problems, second, building resistance through exercise and oxygen intake, and, third, rebuilding through various treatments.

Good things to do for brain health are:

- Eat plants rich in fiber.
- Follow a mild ketogenic diet.
- Twelve- to sixteen hour fasting after your last dinner meal.
- No gluten.
- No simple carbs.
- No dairy.
- Exercise.
- Check your nighttime oxygen intake through an Apple

Watch or other device.

- Reduce excess stress.
- Perform brain training.
- Detox and eat high fiber foods and drink filtered water.
- Include Magnesium and Vitamin D in your diet.
- Increase choline through pasture raised eggs.

Suggested reading: *The First Survivors of Alzheimer's* by Dale Bredesen M.D.

Supplement Suggestions

- Multiple vitamin/mineral
- Essential fatty acids
- Minerals
- Alpha-lipoic acid—50 mg
- Acetyl-L-carnitine—300 mg
- Choline—100-500 mg
- Curcumin-turmeric—400-500 mg
- Mind Power RX herbal brain formula

Inflammation

Chronic inflammation is rapidly becoming a major factor in diseases and in aging. Poor diet, drugs, stress, and toxins all play a role in the formation of inflammation in our bodies. Often inflammation occurs in joints and cartilage for people who have arthritis.

As discussed earlier, testing by biochemical markers c-reactive proteins can measure the amount of inflammation in the body.

Many of the mainstream pharmaceutical anti-inflammatory drugs carry side effects.

Serrapeptase

Serrapeptase, a derivative of the silkworm, has been tested and used in Europe for over ten years with rousing success. This pain relief and anti-inflammatory product is cultivated from silkworms, which use the enzyme to break down the hard shell of their cocoon soon after birth. It has been used in Japan and Europe for over thirty years and is available in prescription form in Austria and Germany. It was introduced into the USA as recently as 2002. German coronary physician Dr. Hans Nieper used serrapeptase to unblock arteries in his heart patients. It dissolved blood clots and caused varicose veins to shrink or diminish. Because it is a natural anti-inflammatory, it can dissolve the dead proteins that bind plaque which can block the arteries, and it supports normal cell growth, joint function, and cardiovascular function.

I have been taking serrapeptase every day as a preventive measure. A woman I know who is in her forties began to take one pill a day and noticed her varicose veins fading in a week's time. Serrapeptase is a natural product that can be taken safely both short- and long-term and will not interfere with other medications. No side effects have been found in any of the vast number of studies and clinical trials. In some cases people have taken thirty capsules a day with no ill effects.

Zyflamend

Another amazing supplement is Zyflamend, a combination of ten herbs for anti-inflammatory and anti-aging. I take it regularly to keep any inflammation away. Zyflamend has been the subject of ongoing research through Columbia University, the Cleveland Clinic, and the MD Anderson Cancer Center.

Supplement Suggestions

- Serrapeptase—dosages vary for various conditions.

- Digestive enzymes and bromelain.
- Nattokinase—helps to dissolve blood clots and lower blood pressure (comes from Japanese soybean).
- ArthroMax—Life Extension formula contains glucosamine sulfate, theaflavins (black tea substance).
- Omega-6 (gamma-linolenic acid).
- Multivitamin/mineral.
- Anti-inflammatory herbs: boswellia (boswellia serrata), turmeric (curcuma longa), ginger (zingiber officinalis).
- Zyflamend.
- Gaia Turmeric Supreme—curcumin-turmeric—400-500 mg.

Immune Conditions

When the immune system is strong, we are protected from antigens (microorganisms, cancer cells, toxins). Antibodies (molecules) are produced to destroy antigens. Autoimmune disease occurs when the immune system is compromised. The body turns on itself and destroys normal body tissues. My mother's RA and lupus were autoimmune diseases.

Vitamin C has long been considered an immune booster because it helps protect cells from free radical damage. Vitamin C intravenous therapy was introduced in the 1950s by Dr. Frederick Klenner. Dr. John Myers did further research on vitamin C IV's and the "Myers's cocktail" was created.

A healthy immune system is influenced by our food choices, stress levels, lifestyles, and airborne toxins. Carotenoids are a type of antioxidant found in green, red, and yellow fruits and vegetables. In a double-blind study, after fifteen days, those who received mixed carotenoids or beta-carotene had significantly less DNA damage than those who did not. In an eight-week study, all groups who received carotenoid supplements showed less DNA damage.

Supplement Suggestions

- Vitamin C or Myers's cocktail
- Glutathione
- Herbs: astragalus, echinacea, garlic, elderberry, cat's claw
- Vitamin E
- Zinc
- Probiotics
- Alpha-lipoic acid

Chemotherapy

Chemicals (antineoplastic) are used in an IV solution to help destroy cancer cells. Unfortunately, besides killing abnormal cells, they also destroy normal cells. My sister had bladder cancer which metastasized into other organs and her brain. I would take her to chemo sessions. Afterward, she would buzz with boundless energy until she crashed. Unfortunately, the treatment made her more ill, and she died within six months. It was a painful process for her and very distressing for our family.

Supplement Suggestions

It is a known fact that all supplements, including vitamins and minerals, are discouraged while a person is on chemotherapy, as they are thought to counteract the effects of the therapy. Until more research can substantially support taking supplements while undergoing chemotherapy, it is advisable to consult with your oncologist.

Research

Unfortunately, new cancer drug research has been bogged down; it may take ten to twenty years for pharmaceutical companies to seek and be awarded patents and FDA approvals. Our antiquated system has prevented more effective therapies from being approved while 1,500 Americans die each day from cancer.

Compassionate Access Act

There is a bill called The Compassionate Access Act of 2010 (H.R. 4732) which was introduced into Congress by The Abigail Alliance, a nonprofit organization. A nineteen-year-old girl, Abigail Burroughs, was diagnosed with squamous cell carcinoma of the neck and lungs. Her oncologist at Johns Hopkins Hospital wanted to use a new drug to help save her life. Unfortunately, this drug hadn't been approved by the FDA even though it showed good responses in early trials. She was ineligible for the drug and after seven months of trying to get approval for its use, she passed away. Sadly, this drug was later approved for use against Abigail's form of cancer. The Compassionate Access Act would amend the Food, Drug, and Cosmetic Act to approve drugs, biological products, and devices for seriously ill patients.

Complementary and Alternative Approaches

Complementary medicine works in complement with conventional medicine—radiation, chemotherapy, and surgery. Alternative medicine uses other methods besides those mentioned. Clinical trial participation is available and eligibility requirements vary. Refer to the resource directory at the end of this book to obtain more information.

Complementary Therapies

- Herbal treatments—ginkgo, ginseng.
- Acupuncture—alleviates nausea.
- Massage—relief from pain, fatigue, depression, and anxiety.

- Yoga—helps strengthen and relax the body.

Alternative Therapies

- 714-X—a cocktail of chemicals that is said to stabilize your immune system so it can fight cancer.
- Essiac—an herbal mixture with supposed antioxidant and anti-inflammatory effects. Refer to the author's book *Essiac: A Native Herbal Cancer Remedy.*
- Gerson therapy—one of several treatments that are said to rid your body of cancer-causing toxins.
- Liver flush—involves the drinking of juices and oils to cleanse the liver of cancer-causing agents.
- Shark cartilage—used to hinder or stop the growth of cancer cells.

Skin Cancer

There are three types of skin cancer: basal cell, squamous, and melanoma, melanoma being the most serious form. Skin cancer is the most easily diagnosed and is primarily due to long unprotected exposure to the sun. Fair-skinned people are especially affected. Between two to three million people are diagnosed with non-melanoma cancer each year. Globally 132,000 melanoma cancers occur each year. According to Skin Cancer Foundation statistics, one in five Americans will get skin cancer.

Cancer and the Sun

Two studies have shown that with the proper amount of vitamin D, risks of developing non-Hodgkin's lymphoma are reduced by 30 to 40 percent. This study included 3,000 lymphoma patients and 3,000 without lymphoma. Also, melanoma patients had less aggressive tumors and less likelihood of dying.

Remember to use common sense when sunbathing: avoid spending hours in the sun, use a natural sunscreen, and stay out of the sun from 10:00 a.m. to 2:00 p.m. As mentioned earlier, Dr. Holick's studies have indicated that vitamin D is only produced during those hours, so supplementing with vitamin D makes sense.

Supplement Suggestions

- Resveratrol.
- Vitamin A.
- Fernblock® supplement which helps shield skin from harmful ultraviolet rays.
- Skin Eternal® by Source Naturals.

High Blood Pressure (Hypertension)

There are two measurements for registering blood pressure: systolic (pressure in arteries when heart beats) and diastolic (heart rests between beats). A normal reading is 120/80. Readings of 140/90 or higher are considered to be high blood pressure. If one has hypertension, heart disease is the number one cause of death. In the US one to three adults have been diagnosed with hypertension. Many more may have high blood pressure but do not know it. Worldwide, one billion people have hypertension. That will rise to 1.56 billion by the year 2025. Factors that play a role in developing hypertension are heredity, aging, obesity, diet, tobacco, and kidney failure (renal insufficiency). In the US, African Americans are at a higher risk than Asians and Caucasians.

Supplement Suggestions

- Coenzyme Q-10.
- Folic Acid—folate is a B vitamin which may help to lower high blood pressure in some people, possibly by reducing elevated homocysteine levels.

- Fish oil—the DHA may help lower blood pressure.
- Hawthorne.
- Garlic—helps reduce systolic and diastolic levels—if taking certain blood thinners, ginkgo, and vitamin E.
- Potassium.
- Magnesium.
- L-arginine.
- Goldenrod.
- Olive leaf.
- Grapeseed.

Low Testosterone

Male Hormones and Testosterone

Testosterone affects most organ systems; it is responsible for facial and body hair and muscle development. It also affects the nervous system, which is linked to aggression and risk-taking. Aging affects testosterone and estrogen levels in men. An enzyme called aromatase is involved in the production of estrogen. It acts by catalyzing the conversion of testosterone (an androgen) to estradiol (an estrogen). Aromatase is found in fat tissue; when men have excessive body fat, it can be an indicator that there is an excess of estrogen levels compared to testosterone.

Some Side Effects of a Decrease in Testosterone

- Depression
- Abdominal fat
- Lowered libido
- Heart disease

- Muscle mass decrease
- High blood pressure
- Diabetes
- Atherosclerosis
- Fatigue

Hormone Testing

After age forty it is suggested that men be tested for both testosterone and estrogen along with having a complete physical exam. It is wise to have multiple testing done over time as hormone levels do vary widely among men. Saliva test kits provided by a certified laboratory will measure estradiol, progesterone, cortisol, testosterone, and DHEA.

Hormone Replacement for Men

There are precautions that should be taken with hormone replacement therapy as there may be contraindications such as the presence of prostate cancer. Certain hormone replacement therapies may contribute to the acceleration of such conditions. Work with a physician for prostate testing and careful monitoring of your hormone therapy.

Therapies to Increase Testosterone

There are many conventional and alternative therapies that a physician may prescribe to increase testosterone levels. They come in various forms: creams, patches, and sublingual tablets. The synthetic forms may produce side effects which could include heart and kidney problems. Athletes have used this type of drugs for better performance and increased muscle mass. These therapies usually require a prescription. Natural therapies prescribed by alternative physicians include creams and sublingual tablets.

Suggested Supplements

- Selenium−200 mcg/day
- Vitamin A−5000 IU/day
- Vitamin E−400 IU/day plus 200 mg of gamma-tocopherol

Several Supplements Are Recommended by Life Extension Foundation to Complement Hormone Therapy.

- Acetyl-L-carnitine—1,000 to 2,000 mg/day
- Chrysin—1,500 mg/day
- Zinc—50 mg/day
- Muira puama—850mg/day
- Quercetin—500 to 1,000 mg/day
- Saw palmetto—320 mg/day
- Nettle root extract—240 mg/day
- DHEA—15 to 75 mg/day with blood testing in three to six weeks

It is strongly suggested that any supplements mentioned here should first be discussed with your physician regarding contraindications and suggested dosages.

Prostate Cancer and Hormones

Studies have revealed that higher levels of testosterone are not linked to prostate enlargement, whereas in older men estradiol (a form of estrogen) produces higher levels of estrogen in the prostate glands and can cause enlargement. Men who already show certain prostate conditions may show an increase in PSA (prostate-specific antigen) levels if on testosterone replacement therapy. If prostate disease has been diagnosed, testosterone therapy is contraindicated as it could cause an increase in cancer cells.

Life Extension Foundation Recommends a Program for Men Which You May Wish to Consider:

- Medical testing which includes blood levels PSA
- Testing free and total testosterone
- Aromatase inhibitors in the case of elevated estrogen levels
- Follow-up testing

The Following Suggestions May Also Be of Benefit:

- Weight loss
- No alcohol (to help liver remove excess estrogen)
- Review all current medications being taken

This information comes from WebMD.com. This site is very useful for researching supplements, benefits, and dosages as well as side effects and interactions.

In Closing

While growing up, sometimes I was asked to retrieve medicine for my parents and grandparents from their bathroom cabinets. I was always so amazed and mystified by the quantity of bottles which contained pills prescribed for various ailments. My mother was very careful not to give us prescriptions or over-the-counter remedies for colds, flu, or other childhood ailments unless it was absolutely necessary. My brother, sister, and I rarely became ill except for my sister's polio scare. My mother's cooking, spending summers at camp, being physically active, and living in a relatively healthy environment all helped. In my junior year in high school, I became sick. I had little energy, found it difficult to breathe, and lacked focus to do most anything. For a couple of weeks, I kept trying to convince my mother that something wasn't quite right with me. She always knew I was a healthy child so had difficulty believing me. Finally, at further insistence she took me to a general doctor who X-rayed my lungs and announced to my mother I had pleurisy, an infection in the lungs. He prescribed bed rest for two weeks. My mother felt so guilty that she hadn't listened to me that she transformed herself into Florence Nightingale during my recuperation period. I slept in her room during the day. She fed me bone marrow soup, broths, and the healthiest foods she could concoct. Naturally, I forgave her and was extremely grateful for her attentiveness.

As my own children had illnesses, I found myself answering a similar call of nursing. I always steered clear of pharmaceutical drugs and treated their childhood illnesses with herbs and various natural remedies. One time my son was taken to our Colorado small town general practitioner with an undiagnosed illness. It seemed serious. The doctor knew almost instantly that my son had encephalitis, a virus which can create acute inflammation of the brain. Trent was hospitalized and came home one week later fully recovered. I recognize that western medicine can play a pivotal role, especially during a crisis situation.

This chapter has covered many health conditions and healthy suggestions. Use your wisdom in making choices when you have an illness, and the true answers will come.

Half the modern drugs could well be thrown out the window, except that the birds might eat them.

—Martin H. Fischer

Step 5

Deeper Than Skin Deep

When I was growing up, we played outside all day. There were no computers or television sets to keep us inside. Our mothers' warnings not to stay out in the sun fell on deaf ears. In college in the late 1950s, sunbathing became a ritual. We slathered on mixtures of baby oil and iodine and baked in the sun. Because of my Italian heritage my olive skin rarely burned, but my fair-skinned friends weren't so fortunate. We never used sunscreen (there was none). What were we thinking? I have read that taking good care of your skin should begin in your twenties—little did we know. As we grow older, perhaps we also grow wiser.

Skin and Your Health

We spend $43 billion annually on over 200 skin care products and cosmetic procedures to make us look better, younger, and healthier. In 2005, North America spent $10 million on cosmetic surgery alone.

Our skin is the largest organ of our bodies. It weighs around ten lb. and covers an area of approximately sixteen square feet. When we overexpose ourselves to sunlight, when we smoke or drink too much alcohol, when our eating habits are unhealthy, it is reflected in the condition of our skin. All these habits contribute to early aging of the skin: wrinkling, sagging, discoloration, and loss of elasticity. The condition of our skin also reflects our internal health.

Mirror, Mirror on the Wall

Have you looked at pictures of yourself when you were younger? I have, and I accept the fact that my hair is grayer, my skin less smooth and firm, and I see more lines. I have tried micro-dermabrasion, facials, and light peels. I have bought creams that guarantee to firm and plump up my sagging skin and lessen wrinkles and lines. Some products seem to bring better results than others, and some are terrifically expensive. I don't recommend the more expensive products because before we use them, we have no way of knowing how really effective they are or how much money we may be wasting.

Even with all the skin care products and wrinkle-smoothing methods out there, good skin care boils down to this: exercise and nutritional programs, attitudes that we have about ourselves, and a choice of products that are free of chemicals and artificial ingredients. Are you positive? Are you stress-free? Do you laugh and fill yourself up with joy? Are you grateful for the good people and experiences in your life? Do you surround yourself with a loving family, partner, and friends? Do you live each day to the fullest? Before bedtime I give thanks for five blessings I have received from my day. It has become a reminder of things I am grateful for. This practice is especially helpful when I have had a challenging day.

From the Inside Out

When we put clean, nutritious, organic (when possible) food into our bodies, our blood delivers healthy nutrients to all of our organs. Dark green leafy vegetables, raw or lightly steamed, help to flush out the toxins that build up in our liver, kidneys, and intestines. When we watch our pH balance (by eating mostly alkaline foods) and exercise properly, the blood pumping through our system provides more strength and endurance, shorter recovery times, and healthier blood cells.

Alcohol consumption, lack of exercise, drugs, acidic foods, and negative attitudes all contribute to harming and compromising our internal organs as well as our largest organ, our skin.

Dry Brushing and Moisturizing the Body

To help detoxify and invigorate your skin, start at your feet and brush toward your heart with a natural bristle brush. I enjoy dry brushing with a natural loofah-type brush before my shower and applying pure virgin coconut oil on my body, including my face and hair. Coconut oil is not only versatile in cooking, but applied topically it increases metabolism, heals injuries, and helps to smooth and firm the skin.

Pure virgin coconut oil is high in antioxidants that penetrate into the underlying tissues of our skin to prevent and protect against the formation of free radicals (which break down the skin's connective tissues as we age). The oil will also soften and moisturize skin while removing the outer layer of dead skin cells, making your skin smoother and more evenly textured with a healthy "shine." Be careful when purchasing body oils and lotions; many conventional body care products made with refined vegetable oils have all the antioxidants stripped from them (as a result of the refining process) and so are highly prone to free radical generation, causing your skin to actually age faster.

Factors That Promote Early Aging and Wrinkling of the Skin

- Smoking
- Skin type (people with light skin and blue eyes are more susceptible to sun damage)
- Heredity
- Occupational and recreational sun exposure over the course of many years
- Weight fluctuations
- Dehydration
- Lack of proper nutrients; essential fatty acids (fishtail or flaxseed oil)
- Poor diet: processed foods and low in plant foods
- Lack of exercise
- Stress

- Inadequate sleep
- Chemicals and drugs
- Toxins, hormone decline, inflammation toxins, elevated glucose levels—sugars bind to collagen creating sagging and wrinkles

Shower Filters

Our skin is the largest organ of our body, so just like water filters for drinking, showering, and bathing with filters protects our skin from heavy metals, copper, and chlorine. A good shower filter balances our PH, improves our skin and hair, removes scaling from the shower and softens our skin. There are many excellent products available; Culligan RDSHC115, Jonathan Product Beauty Shower, Waterchef SF-7C, Aquasana AQ4100, Culligan WSH-C125.

These filters are easy to install, and the filter should be replaced every six months. I purchase these on Amazon.

Tip: Take warm and then cool shower for brief time to avoid toxins and drying out skin. Never use an antibacterial soap. They contain triclosan, which has not proven to be effective and may be harmful.

Skin Care Basics

The main preventive measures to help us maintain a healthy body (both internally and externally) are minimize excessive sun exposure; don't smoke; eat healthy foods; drink plenty of filtered water; reduce stress; and take antioxidants. We know that overexposure to the sun's UVB rays can damage the collagen and elastic fibers in the skin and create liver spots, wrinkles, rough, and sagging skin—especially if we have spent years in the sun.

Sunscreens

The first true sunscreens came on the market in the early 1970s. The leading ingredient, PABA, was favored for binding readily to cells and for its water resistance. However, many people found it stained their clothing and some developed allergic reactions to this ingredient. It was later discovered that PABA may have been damaging to DNA. Obviously, few products today contain PABA, but we do have some smart choices of brands that are most beneficial and kinder to our older skin.

Safely Using Sunscreens

There has been some controversy about sunscreens. Are they safe to use and what kinds of sunscreens are better than others?

A majority of the sunscreens in the marketplace today contain one or more of the chemicals octyl-methoxycinnamate (OMC), quaternium 15, DMDM hydantoin, and parabens. A study performed at the Norwegian Radiation Protection Authority in Oslo showed that when the tissue culture of mice was exposed to a solution of OMC (far less than contained in sunscreens), it caused 50 percent of the cells to die, and when exposed to a sunlamp for two hours, more cells died, making the effect twice as toxic. When a sunscreen's purpose is to be used in the sun, what does that tell us about the safety of OMC?

Other Chemicals Besides OMC to Look Out For

- Benzophenone-3 (Bp-3)
- Homosalate (HMS)
- 4-methyl-benzylidene camphor (4-MBC)
- Octyl-dimethyl-PABA (OD-PABA)
- Octyl-methoxycinnamate
- Parabens (butyl-, ethyl-, methyl-, and propyl)

These chemicals are considered estrogenic, meaning any of several steroid hormones produced chiefly by the ovaries are responsible for promoting estrus and the development and maintenance of female secondary sex characteristics. They fool the body into believing they are naturally produced hormones.

Two vital hormones that help to protect our skin are DHEA and melatonin. DHEA is an anti-stress hormone that helps safeguard against tissue destruction and accelerated aging by transporting essential nutrients through the blood stream. Topical use of DHEA performs 85 to 90 percent better than through supplementation. Melatonin is a sleep hormone and a free radical scavenger that enhances the skin's ability to repair free radical damage.

Sun Creams

I prefer going the chemical-free route in skin products; I find the more natural sunscreens much less irritating to my skin. I try not to put chemicals in my body, so why should I put them *on* my body, since the skin is the body's largest organ.

Here is a partial list of some sun products that are more beneficial and much kinder for your skin. Look for a natural sunscreen that protects from UVA (aging) and UVB (burning) rays with an SPF of at least 15 up to 30 SPF and use it year-around. These brands can often be found in your local health food store.

- Aubrey Organics® has an SPF 18 and 30 and Ultra Natural
- Herbal Sun Block
- Kiss My Face®, SPF 18 and 30
- Bronzo Sensuale®, SPF 30
- Lavera® (zinc oxide and titanium dioxide)
- Devita Daily Solar Protective Moisturizer ® (zinc oxide)
- Epicuren Discovery Zinc Oxide Sunscreen®
- JASON Naturals Sunbrellas Chemical-Free Sunblock® (zinc oxide and titanium dioxide)
- Goddess Garden
- Badger

- Seventh Generation Derma E

All of these products are biodegradable. Most of these products contain similar ingredients: vitamins, antioxidants, shea butter, aloe vera, sesame oil, avocado oil, lanolin, zinc oxide, titanium dioxide (protects against UVA and UVB rays), and green tea (shown to protect against skin cancer)

In addition to putting sun creams on your skin, antioxidants will increase the body's ability to handle sun without burning. Astaxanthin is a powerful antioxidant that can be purchased at health food stores and is also found in shrimp, crawfish, lobster, and crab. It is an internal sunscreen that allows you to stay in the sun twice as long. Include vitamin C, green tea extract, or whole grape extract in your diet, and vitamin E lotion or pure vitamin E on your skin. Proper nutrition and plenty of pure water for hydration helps to keep the skin healthy.

Sun Tips

- Avoid burning.

- Limit your sun exposure by staying out of the sun between 10:00 a.m. and 2:00 p.m.

- Allow sun exposure no more than two to three times weekly If you are not used to being in the sun, gradually build up your exposure beginning with fifteen minutes a day and slowly increasing your time in the sun; fair-skinned people have a tendency to burn more easily because of the lower amount of melanin; I have been blessed with olive skin and tan easily.

- Wear clothing that shields the sun's rays from the skin, or simply wear a long-sleeve shirt, long pants or skirt, hat, and sunglasses.

- People with dark pigmentation may actually tolerate twenty to thirty times more sun exposure than their fair-skinned counterparts.

Skin Treatments

Skin treatments can be confusing; there are so many being touted as the best for eliminating wrinkles, firming the epidermis, and boosting levels of collagen (a protein that works with elastin to give the body its tone and suppleness) that it's hard to sort it all out.

Treatments available for wrinkles include retinol (vitamin A), alpha hydroxy acids, antioxidants, lipid-based serums, and moisturizers. Medical cosmetic procedures include glycolic acid peels, deep peels, microdermabrasion, laser resurfacing, surgical procedures (facelifts), Botox® injections, laser treatments, and a multitude of new skin treatment choices which seem to appear daily. Of course, if you want to go all the way, cosmetic surgeons are always there. Take the time to find a reputable, board-certified cosmetic surgeon if surgery is in your future.

Facial Rejuvenation Acupuncture

While living in Hawaii I participated in a free session with several acupuncturists who were being taught how to apply needles on the face for rejuvenation. After the painless treatment, I decided to sign up for twelve weekly sessions with a locally trained acupuncturist to experience how my skin would improve in a healthier manner rather than submitting to cosmetic surgery procedures. Initially, the acupuncturist did a TCM (traditional Chinese medicine) diagnosis which is done by checking the pulse, the tongue, and by observation. Not only were the sessions relaxing, but I also noticed my age spots lightening and my skin becoming rosier in color and feeling firmer.

Based on the principles of TCM, acupuncture increases circulation throughout the blood and lymph system. Facial acupuncture helps the whole body look and feel younger by addressing the physical, mental, and emotional patterns that cause disease and contribute to the aging process. Our skin ages for a number of reasons besides sun exposure: unhealthy diet, worry, overwork—all of which contribute to a depleted spleen, poor digestion, and chronic infections. The health of our internal organs is also reflected in our outer appearance. For instance, if our kidneys are depleted, our bones and head are affected. Dark circles under our eyes may indicate a kidney imbalance. Dull skin indicates poor elimination.

While thousands of herbal formulations have been created throughout the 2,000-year history of acupuncture, few can equal the benefits of this ancient practice. Acupuncture is a very old science resulting in very youthful results.

There is an exact science with Chinese medicine. I would suggest studying up on this illuminating and fascinating subject.

The Treatment

Extremely fine needles are inserted into specific areas of the face. The entire procedure is relaxing and is usually done two times weekly in twenty-to-thirty-minute sessions.

Benefits of Facial Acupuncture:

- Eliminates fine lines and diminishes wrinkles.
- Improves muscle tone and dermal contraction and tightens pores.
- Increases collagen production.
- Eliminates and reduces bags under the eyes and lifts drooping eyelids.
- Decreases sagging.
- Reduces or eliminates double chins.
- Eliminates puffiness.
- Improves skin color.

- Brightens the eyes.
- Reduces stress evident in the face.
- Enhances innate beauty and radiance.

Precautions

If you are pregnant or experiencing allergic reactions, have herpes, a cold or the flu, wait until the symptoms subside and consult with the practitioner before initiating sessions. This treatment may not be for you if severe conditions exist such as high blood pressure or diabetes, or if you are using anticoagulants including aspirin or coumadin®. If you have had recent laser resurfacing or microdermabrasion, allow one to three months before facial acupuncture treatments.

Ion-Photon-Sonic Machine

- Ultra renew plus

  This FDA-approved anti-aging device uses ultrasonic technology using three different light therapies. Red light—reduces breakouts, reduces broken capillaries, reduces crow's feet, reduces fine lines, reduces redness, reduces wrinkles, rosacea-friendly, safe to use on areas treated with fillers, suitable for sensitive skin types, tightens skin. Blue light—boosts collagen production, boosts elastin production, boosts radiance, clinically tested, evens skin tone. Green light—hyper pigmentation, reduces brown spots.

This product can be used as often as you wish. Each session can be as short as seven to ten minutes. The ultra renew kit includes the machine, glasses, and instructions. You can also purchase an aloe vera gel which is used directly on your clean skin. The gel helps the machine to move comfortably. The machine can be purchased on Amazon.

Facial Massage—Creating Youthful Skin

There are forty-two muscles in our face. We use these muscles for four basic facial expressions. Facial muscles, along with the head and neck muscles, need to be relaxed so they can stretch and contract at a healthy level. We exercise our bodies, so why not our faces?

When muscle isn't used, it shrinks. Skin can handle pressure. You can do facial massage every day and once you learn the techniques, it only takes ten minutes. To perform facial exercises, your skin needs to be clean and free of makeup. The areas to massage include the forehead, eyes, nose, cheeks, jaw, and neck. There are many techniques demonstrated on YouTube as well as on DVDs that can be purchased online. You can apply a thin layer of an essential oil such as lavender, argon, jojoba, coconut, frankincense, evening primrose, or rosehip oils if you desire. Essential oils are very beneficial and healthy for the skin. Remember to rub upward so you don't drag your skin down.

You can massage each area fifty times and may build up to 100, 150, and 200.

Benefits

- Eliminates wrinkles.
- Lifts face.
- Adds rosy complexion.
- Drains lymph system.
- Contours and shapes face back to your 20s.
- Improves elasticity.
- Removes toxins.
- Reduces dark circles and puffy skin.
- Removes jowls and sagging neck.

This information comes from www.cynthiarowland.com.

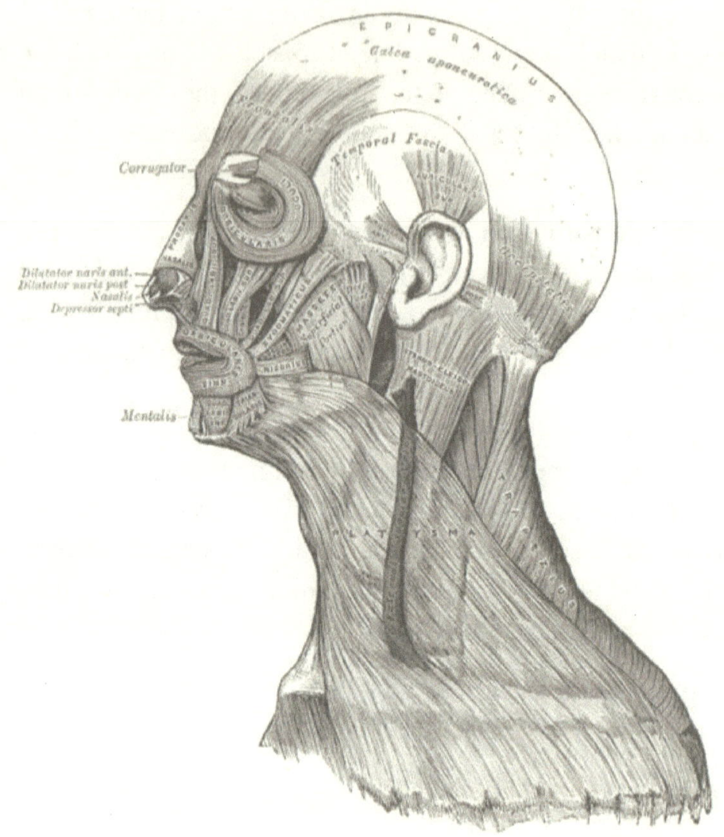

Acupressure Points

There are acupressure points throughout your body. If you use acupressure on your face, it helps to relieve stress from your face and effect meridians, which benefit different organs. Take your finger and make small circles for each point starting with one minute and you can gradually build up to a few minutes. Start with your chin and work yourself upward.

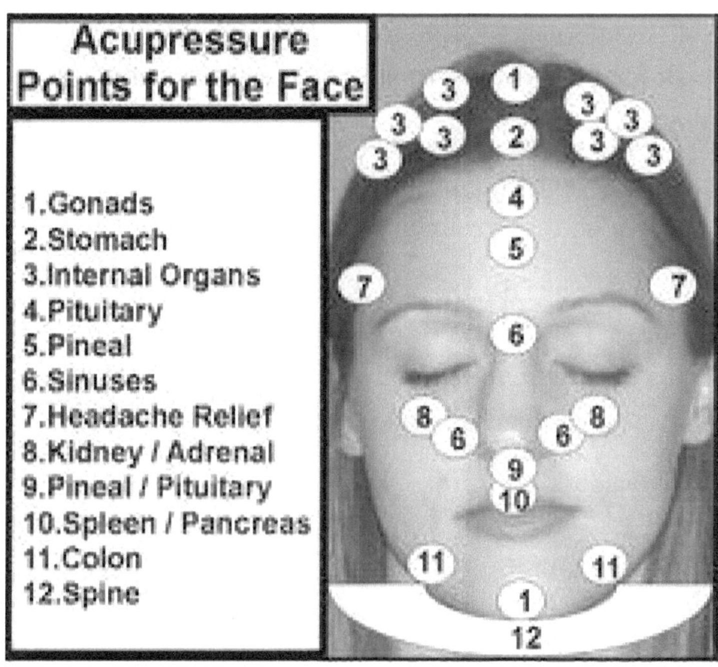

Suggestions on How to Clean the Face

In the morning, splash warm water over your face several times. Follow by splashing cold water on your face to close pores. Apply your day cream and sun cream. In the evening, wash your face with a mild soap or natural face wash. Use warm water followed by cold water. Then apply your nighttime cream.

Black and Brown Spots

Excessive production of melanin can produce dark pigmentation on the face and body. Hormonal shifts, sunbathing, and stress also contribute to dark spots. Following are simple ways to reduce pigmentation without using chemical ingredients. Be patient as the results may take several weeks to notice.

- Apple cider vinegar and water—use equal amounts of vinegar and water and let it sit on skin for ten minutes. Rinse and repeat in evening.

- Lemon-honey and olive oil—Add equal amounts and let it sit for ten minutes. Rinse and repeat in evening.
- Turmeric and lemon juice—Add equal amounts and let it sit for twenty minutes. Rinse with cool water. Avoid sun for one hour after treatment.
- Aloe Vera and honey—two tsp. aloe vera gel and half tsp. honey. Let it sit on skin for ten minutes then apply on skin for twenty minutes. Rinse with warm water. May be used once a day for two weeks, then every other day.
- Avocado-honey-milk—mash one avocado, two tsp. honey, one tsp. milk. Allow to dry, then rinse. Do this once a day for one month.

This information comes from www.top10homeremedies.com.

Dry Facial Brushes

Face brushes can be used to stimulate blood flow, activate the lymphatic system, and rid the face of dead skin cells. Follow with a facial massage with facial oil.

Derma Roller

This is a device with micro needles on it. If you order a derma roller, the .50 ml is minimum needle size to boost collagen production. This is a popular size and can be used two to three times a week. The .75 ml to 1 ml derma roller can be used every two weeks. The 1.5 ml to 3 ml size can cause severe scaring and should only be used once per month. Otherwise, it could damage your skin. You will need at least three months to see improvement to your skin. You do not need to apply anything on the clean skin to use the roller. I use mine at night because it makes my skin red. A derma roller causes thousands of needle punctures in the skin; therefore, it is not advisable to believe people on the web who make claims that are different.

You can pull your skin to help the needles penetrate better. A derma roller should not be used to treat acne. It can spread acne. Do not use 5 ml and above to treat acne. After use, put your roller in a cup with alcohol and leave for ten to fifteen minutes. If you have very sensitive skin, apply numbing cream and wait thirty minutes before doing the treatment. Roll three to four times up and down, across and diagonally each way. You may use the other hand to stretch your skin taut. You can have a smaller roller head to get into areas that are more difficult to get to. Use vitamin C serum after your session.

Benefits

- Boosts collagen and elastin production.
- Prevents premature aging.
- Reduces hyperpigmentation and UV damage.
- Reduces large pores.
- Reduces rough skin.
- Boosts serum and cream absorption.

Skin Care for Mature Skin

As we age, our skin becomes increasingly rough and wrinkled and may show some irregular pigmentation (coloration). All this is due to the natural decrease in our body's production of collagen and elastin. Our skin requires different care with age. As we grow older, our skin doesn't produce new cells at the same pace. Environmental and biological factors take their toll. We often develop enlarged pores, and the effects of the sun become evident in age spots, wrinkles, and freckles. Our desire is to replenish dry, sensitive, and aging skin in the most beneficial method made available.

There are a staggering 1,000-plus chemicals and preservatives that you want to avoid, and many of them are present in mainstream over-the-counter cosmetic and skin care products. In 2003 the European Commission banned most of these chemicals from beauty products. In the US, the Food and Drug Administration (FDA) has lagged behind, only banning nine of the hundreds of chemicals from cosmetic products. There is, however, a website you can access for information on companies who have signed a pledge not to use the European-banned chemicals. Remember, our skin is the largest organ in the body and absorbs everything we put on it; it seems to make sense to use the freshest and most pure ingredients possible, doesn't it?

Skin Lines

- MyChelle Dermaceuticals®
- Juice Beauty® certified organics
- Dr. Hauschka
- Yes to
- Zia Naturals
- Life Extension skin
- Acure
- Welled
- Galen's Way
- Argonne
- Josie Maran
- Origins
- Trilipiderm Caudalie

Not all products are 100 percent organic, and the industry is unregulated. The best way to decide is to read the labels and consult with professionals who recommend products that do not contain harmful chemicals.

Chemicals to Avoid

- Coal Tar
- Formaldehyde
- DEA/TEA/MEA
- Fragrance/Parfum
- Ethoxylated surfactants and 1,4-dioxane
- Mercury
- Lead
- Parabens
- Hydroquinone
- Phthalates
- Polyethylene glycol (PEG)
- Silicone-derived emollients
- Sodium lauryl sulfate
- Talc
- Toluene Triclosan

This information comes from treehugger.com.

Suggested book by Gillian Deacon, *There's Lead in your Lipstick: Toxins in Our Everyday Body Care and How to Avoid Them*

Makeup

There are so many makeup lines out there that a woman could lose her mind deciding which ones to buy. For the sake of simplicity, I am listing some of the mineral makeup lines that are natural as well as available online and in health stores.

- Mineral Makeup

- Jane Iredale
- Youngblood
- English Mineral
- bareMinerals
- Bobbi Brown
- Lily Lolo
- Josie Maran
- Laura Mercier

Hyaluronic Acid

This product helps to capture water molecules, diminish wrinkles, and combat free radicals A new, more effective modified hyaluronic acid product tested by Rutgers University shows an increase in moisture to the skin six times more than regular hyaluronic acid and its effects last for twenty-four hours (lifeextension.com).

Exfoliating

Exfoliating skin daily helps cellular turnover, stimulates collagen, and removes dry skin, which prepares the skin for a water-base serum and moisturizing cream with an SPF of 30. Avoid petroleum and lanolin ingredients as they clog the skin. I discovered a 2 percent retinol serum at the health store which I apply once daily, usually at night. I also use a vitamin C serum with 28 percent concentrate each morning before applying my moisturizer and sunscreen. Twice monthly, I apply a 50 percent lactic acid peel. It is wise to start with a lower percentage and gradually build up until your skin becomes adjusted. This helps with cellular turnover and exposes newer, fresher, more youthful skin. I wash with a Clarisonic® brush which cleans the face using a micro-massage action. According to clinical studies, when used properly it removes makeup six times better than manual facial cleansing, cleans pores, and makes skin products more absorbable and effective.

There are myriads of wonderful skin creams available. Explore, research, and discover how you can have healthier, more radiant, and youthful looking skin without paying a premium price. Find out which ones work for your particular skin type. I suggest you find a local aesthetician that you trust to help you decide which treatments and products are best for you.

If you are fortunate enough to live in a moist climate rather than a dryer high-altitude or desert climate, your skin can feel like velvet. If you do live in a dry climate, use a humidifier, and frequently mist and moisturize your skin. Remember to drink plenty of filtered water, limit sun exposure between the hours of 10:00 a.m. and 2:00 p.m., use a safe sunscreen every day, and most of all be happy and enjoy your life!

Spas: More Than Skin Deep

A weekend at a spa could easily cost $500 or more for lodging, meals, a few treatments, and perhaps a class or two. Spa-goers want more than just the massage experience. We want advice on how to maintain and improve our skin through products, nutrition, and techniques that we can use in our own homes.

Coconut Skin Wash Recipe

- One cup organic coconut oil
- 1/8 cup baking soda
- 5 drops lavender oil
- 5 drops frankincense oil

Heat coconut oil and then let cool. Add other ingredients and let sit until firm. Put in glass container and store in bathroom. Wash face daily with the coconut mixture. This will keep your skin healthy and moisturized.

Homemade Facial Toner

After cleaning morning and evening, I apply a small amount of toner over my skin. Results have been diminished dark spots, smaller pores, and healthier skin.

Two ounces Bretanna witch hazel infused germanium rose hip and aloe essential oils, two ounces jojoba oil, and five drops grapefruit oil.

The Perfect Spa in Your Own Home

You can treat yourself to a spa day in the comfort of your own home. Begin your day with silence and a stretch. Soak in a lavender-scented bath—a great stress reliever. Adding sea salts also helps to detoxify the body. Light candles and turn off the phone. Give yourself a facial by blending oatmeal and milk in a blender to make a paste and apply it to your clean face. This mask helps to draw out toxins and increase circulation. Soak two steeped chamomile tea bags in ice-cold milk and place on eyelids for ten minutes to reduce puffiness and rejuvenate tired eyes. Eat light and healthy foods. Take a walk. Read a book or watch a funny movie.

The information in this section is intended to act only as a guide. Each of us has our own skin type, our own lifestyles and our own attitudes. Do not try to compare yourself to friends, strangers, or models in magazines. Do not be too easily influenced by "miracle" anti-aging medical procedures. Create your own identity and be a most beautiful, compassionate friend to yourself.

Step 6

Take Charge of Your Finances: Health and Home

How I Developed Passion for a Healthy Lifestyle

As you know, I watched my mother suffer from rheumatoid arthritis (an autoimmune disease) while I was growing up and saw that none of the prescriptions she was given for her pain and swelling fifty years ago helped to improve her debilitating disease. While I was in college, I received a phone call from my mother. She had fallen while getting out of her tub, had snapped her hip, and was in the hospital awaiting surgery. She was forty-five at the time. She tried to explain to me what had happened; however, the medications and the fall were causing hallucinations—she said there were creatures under her hospital bed, and she was frightened and couldn't understand why she was in the hospital. After trying to soothe her, I called my family and demanded to know why I wasn't told my mother was in the hospital. The response was "we didn't want to worry you." This was the standard line for various family situations that arose.

After hip surgery, my mother refused physical therapy and never walked again. She later contracted lupus, had a stroke, and passed away at fifty-two years of age. My father, who was nine years older, had been her caregiver. As a family we were never informed of his own blood disorder. My father was a very private man and never discussed his health with his children. My parents passed away within six weeks of one another. I felt a profound sense of loss—especially because they had died so young. There were never any preventive or alternative treatments considered for my parents during that time. The prescribed drugs may have eased my mother's severe pain and joint swelling, but the side effects created severe depression and I believe eventually led to the onset of lupus and premature death.

Thus, in my midtwenties, after my parents' passing, I began my quest for alternative healing. All these years later I continue along my path of well-being through Chinese doctors, regular massages, and contacting a naturopathic doctor in my area if certain health conditions arise. I do not take prescription drugs unless it is absolutely necessary. I prefer complementary medicine and have for many years. I have changed my nutritional habits throughout the years, continue to exercise, and pursue core strengthening activities such as yoga, Pilates, and dance. I manage the stress of everyday living through breath work, meditation, and gratitude for the blessings I receive each day. Today's medicine and healing has come a long way since my parents' time.

The New Medicine

PBS aired a documentary in March of 2006 entitled *The New Medicine*. The show was hosted by Dana Reeve, who was later diagnosed with lung cancer following the death of her actor husband, Christopher Reeve. Sadly, Dana passed away shortly after her husband's death, although reports stated she was not a cigarette smoker.

The show focused on mainstream, traditional doctors and medical departments not known for being "cutting edge" or "alternative/complementary." The cameras went into health-care clinics, private practices, and research institutions to illustrate a new movement taking place in medical clinics and hospitals around the country; to treat the patient as a whole person and consider, among other things, their lifestyle, culture, and stress factors.

The medical community is beginning to recognize the importance of their patients' desires to get well and place more emphasis on prevention rather than treating a patient with a disease-based protocol. Many hospitals are integrating complementary modalities like acupuncture into their systems. The Latin root word for doctor means teacher. A proactive physician can help a patient avoid disease by teaching them how to take better care of themselves through preventive measures. This progressive outlook presents a new medical paradigm in health care and prevention of disease. Since 1948, the United Nations World Health Organization definition of health has been an active "state of complete physical, mental and social well-being."

This information comes from www.who.int.

A new era in preventive medicine has emerged. Founded in 1995, the World Academy of Anti-Aging and Regenerative Medicine (WAAM) makes available to physicians (MDs) and osteopaths (DOs) fellowships, extensive course training, and studies in age management and regenerative medicine. This knowledge is also available to institutions, researchers, and accredited universities throughout the world. Understanding how cells function and regenerate tissues and organs can represent a revolutionary breakthrough for people around the globe. Age management consists of individualized evaluations and testing which include hormone levels, nutrition, brain cognitive testing, and physical performance. Through physical exams and performance testing, these customized programs can assist in improving one or more of the following conditions or symptoms: excess weight, lack of muscle tone, low libido, hormonal imbalances, and impaired cognitive processes.

Regenerative Medicine

Wake Forest University Baptist Institute for Regenerative Medicine, created in 2004, offers new medical research and leading-edge bioengineering. This is the largest facility in the world in its field; it has more than 150 scientists devoting their expertise toward developing organs for transplant into the bodies of people. These organs range from bladders to heart valves and arteries. The blood and the cells of the patients are placed into a mold of the organ or body part and incubated. Anthony Atala, MD, the director of the institute, has had long-term success and improvement in the lives of children and teenagers who have received new bladders from these advanced procedures. My sister was diagnosed with bladder cancer and at the time, the doctor's answer was to remove her bladder. She refused because she was adamant that she would not carry around an ostomy bag for the remainder of her life.

Stem Cell Definition

Stem Cells: One of the human body's master cells, with the ability to grow into any one of the body's more than 200 cell types.

All stem cells are unspecialized (undifferentiated) cells that are characteristically of the same family type (lineage). They retain the ability to divide throughout life and give rise to cells that can become highly specialized and take the place of cells that die or are lost.

Stem cells contribute to the body's ability to renew and repair its tissues. Unlike mature cells, which are permanently committed to their fate, stem cells can both renew themselves and create new cells of whatever tissue they belong to (and other tissues).

This information comes from medicinenet.com.

Stem Cell Therapy Around the World

Countries that practice stem cell therapies vary in their funding, religion, and embryonic approaches.

The UK, Canada, United States, European Union (EU), South Korea, Australia, Switzerland, Spain, and Mexico are a few of the countries that are active in stem cell therapies, although they all vary. Germany, Austria, and Italy are much stricter in their stem cell protocols.

It is best to research. Because not all information is reputable, I have included some that I trust.

- https://the-stem-cell-center.com/Stem-Cell-Therapy?msclkid=824e222609d91cf13cb54206a08716a0&msclkid=c7dca1d798df136a6f11c20fbc7e1ffa

- Department of Health: http://www.dh.gov.uk
- UK National Stem Cell Network: http://www.uknscn.org
- Medical Research Council: http://www.mrc.ac.uk
- International Society For Stem Cell Research: http://www.isscr.org

Books published after 2000:

- *Proteus Effect: Stem Cells and Their Promise in Medicine*
- *Parkinson's Disease: A Complete Guide for Patients and Families*
- *Bone Marrow and Blood Stem Cell Transplants: A Guide for Patients*
- *The Human Cloning Debate*
- *Understanding DNA and Gene Cloning: A Guide for the Curious*

Updated research and studies can be found on:

- https://www.sciencedaily.com/news/health_medicine/stem_cells/
- http://www.ncbi.nlm.nih.gov/pmc/articles/PMC2744936/

Stanford University Stem Cell Replacement

According to the *Science Translational Medicine* journal, thousands of people may be assured of safe and effective stem cell replacements for arthritis, diabetes, multiple sclerosis, and lupus thanks to medical research at Stanford University. Autoimmune disease attacks its own body. Doctors have found that by using bone marrow cells from healthy people, it can reset the immune system and avoid near fatal results. So far, the testing has only been done on animals. "If it works in humans like it did in mice, we would expect that the risk of death from blood stem cell transplant would drop from 20 percent to effectively zero," says Dr. Judith Shizuru, professor of medicine at Stanford (Vaughan, 2016).

The chemotherapy and radiation used for transplant damage DNA and can cause both immediate problems and long-term damage to many tissues in the body. "Among the many known toxic side effects, these treatments can cause damage to the liver, reproductive organs, and brain, potentially causing seizures and impairing neurological development and growth in children," says Dr. Shizuru.

The scientists have developed antibodies, which attach to the damaged stem cells, which get flushed away. This would allow for the new stem cell process to generate new blood and a healthy immune system. Currently, patients who receive stem cell surgery are required to stay on medicine for the remainder of their life.

Hyperbaric Chamber

I read that the performer Michael Jackson had his own hyperbaric chamber. If we could all afford to have one, we might be healthier for it. The pressure in a hyperbaric chamber causes the oxygen to dissolve into all of the body fluids so that the red blood cells and blood plasma become drenched with oxygen. Plasma carries extra oxygen to areas where circulation is poor or blocked, by trickling past the blockages or by seeping into the areas that the red blood cells are too large to reach. Plasma is made up of smaller particles than red blood cells. This extra oxygen provides the extra energy needed in the healing process. New capillaries are formed which aid in healing wounds, autism, brain function, cerebral palsy, poor circulation, and gangrene to name a few.

Dr. Edgar End was most prominent and knowledgeable on hyperbaric benefits as a clinical professor of environmental medicine at the University of Wisconsin Medical School. He noted: "I've seen partially paralyzed people half carried into the (HBOT) chamber, and they walk out after the first treatment. If we got to these people quickly, we could prevent a great deal of damage."

A person lies in the pressurized glassed chamber which provides a 360-degree view. The treatment lasts up to an hour, and there may be music or even television provided. There are solo hyperbaric chambers, chambers that hold two people, and group chambers. If you are interested, you can do a little research in your area to see what is available.

Infrared Saunas

While living in Hawaii, I was most fortunate to often be able to use an infrared sauna. It was situated on some property owned by a woman who had a small natural healing center. The sauna was located outside. The unit contained several fiberglass carbon infrared heaters, a bench, and windows. I would sit inside for twenty to thirty minutes allowing the heat to absorb into my body. I was able to control the temperature from inside. Research indicates heat can absorb more than 1.5 inches into the body. Sitting in the sauna can help reduce toxins and help burn the calories equivalent to running two to three miles. After my session I would walk a few feet to a lovely Hawaiian outdoor shower area to rinse off, feeling refreshed and energized.

The Healing Machine

While wandering the downtown streets of San Clemente, California, I spotted a sign that read "Health Center." In the store I was introduced to a space-age looking machine called Turbosonic®. It was developed, patented, and introduced in Germany. After decades of research and development, the machines are now in the US with FDA approval. A person stands on a platform while receiving sonic vibrations at different frequencies. Various levels of vibration can be set to improve medical conditions such as emphysema, osteoporosis, arthritis and rheumatism, multiple sclerosis, and lower back pain. Results are felt in as little as ten minutes on the machine. It replaces an hour and half of conventional exercise for muscle development, core conditioning, and weight loss. It increases cellular oxygen circulation while moving cellular waste out of the body. Other benefits include improved balance, coordination, and flexibility. I experienced lower back pain on my road trip from Colorado to California. In one session my back pain disappeared, I felt more energized during the day, and I slept soundly at night. To access in-depth studies, refer to the resources at the back of this book.

Taking Steps toward Improved Health

How can you actively participate in addressing your health concerns as well as implement preventive steps for a long and healthy life? You can contact WAAM or locate a practitioner in your area who may be recommended by a friend or another wellness professional. Continue to educate yourself about alternative and complementary procedures through the excellent magazines, books, and web resources available. Massage, acupuncture, herbs, and infrared saunas are only a few of the modalities available today that help to complement your whole picture of health and vitality. Find a health practitioner whom you trust. Locate physicians who are educating themselves in different healing modalities to supplement traditional medical care and the customary reliance on prescription pharmaceuticals. Acupuncture and massage therapy help treat such conditions as back pain or stress-related illnesses and can be far less expensive through an alternative practitioner.

Steps to Your Financial Future

I grew up in a conservative East Coast family. My father was an engineer who received a free college scholarship at Cooper Union College in New York City. My mother had a business degree, and my grandfather was a college graduate from Italy. My grandmother quit school after eighth grade and worked to support her Italian mother who did not speak English. She lived with my grandparents helping to raise her two daughters, my mother, and my aunt. My grandfather's first wife had died after giving birth to my aunt. She was not able to read or write well nor did she ever drive a car. Her husband, on the other hand, was a graduate of New York University. His father had died at an early age leaving his wife to raise a number of children, many of whom were able to work their way through college.

My Italian grandparents were an enterprising couple who developed a plastics company in 1918 in the US, and their hard work over the next thirty-five years provided them a comfortable life. We could have lived in large, elegant homes, driven expensive cars, worn expensive clothes and jewelry, and traveled around the world, but my family did not believe in spending money on possessions. As young adults my brother, sister, and I didn't expect to live in the lap of luxury. We were happy. My parents' idea of redecorating wasn't buying new furniture and "things" for our home but to put the winter drapes away and hang the lighter summer ones and put summer slipcovers on the living room furniture. Because my father was an engineer, he was a master at fixing broken things. (He remodeled a section of the basement as our play area.)

Our Christmas gifts were ice skates, sleds, mittens, clothes, a new bike, and a few toys. We had two cars for my parents, but I rode my bicycle to school every day. We saved money for necessities like doctor and dental checkups, school, food, and clothing. We had a freezer which held meats and poultry. Food didn't spoil and get thrown away. We didn't have a dishwasher, so after each evening meal my sister and I would wash and dry dishes. My brother sometimes managed to sneak off before putting them away. My sister and I shared a bedroom which was a converted attic. We held down summer jobs during high school, were fortunate to be given college educations, and were taught values and principles. My parents and grandparents always lived within their means. They only bought homes without mortgages and while some of our friends' parents were spending beyond their resources and in debt, we lived without any fear of collapse. My grandparents donated money to colleges, hospitals, and an orphanage in the Italian town where my grandfather grew up. My grandfather didn't invest in the stock market but chose instead to develop and invest in real estate, which brought him great rewards. It was a period in life when people were enterprising, worked hard, and were practical. Families were of primary importance. To this day I detest excess or waste in my life.

My Career Challenges

Carolyn Myss is an international author and speaker who has an interesting take on job descriptions during our lifetimes. In our earlier years Carolyn's belief is that our work is called a "job." Perhaps as a college graduate, we are testing the deeper waters outside the classroom. My first job after college was as an elementary school teacher. I was following my major as an educator, but it fell short of my expectations in a short time. Following that brief experience, I took a humdrum job in a credit bureau office in Washington DC where my organization and people skills were finely honed. I was paid more than the other girls just because I had a college diploma.

During the 1950s and 1960s many women were expected to attend college, get married, have children, and become homemakers similar to Julie Robert's depiction of a 1950s college teacher in the movie *Mona Lisa Smile*. While in my twenties, my husband and family moved to Snowmass, Colorado. I purchased my first affordable retail business which was a small kitchen shop in the middle of a mountain village. Shortly after that, my sister-in-law became my business partner. During the next four years, I learned about buying items, displaying, and managing finances. Then suddenly, a messy and traumatic divorce forced me to sell my business and move. Today, looking back on that pivotal time in my life, being a single mother of three young children, I remember feeling rocked to the core and that I had very little worth or self-esteem. I was in my early thirties and inexperienced in coping with this major episode I never anticipated.

My decision to remarry a year later was built on my still rocky foundation and feelings of desertion stemming from my previous marriage. My second husband had custody of his two young boys. My world was tilting left and right with five small children ranging in age from four to ten to take care of. During the next eight years I held part-time jobs to help provide a more even keel and balance between the multitude of motherly duties in a full house, finding me among all of the activity, and making the marriage work. Alcoholism tore the relationship apart, and once again I took the next steps into the void.

However, this time was different. My children were older; I was braver and more self-assured. I was also grateful that my parents weren't still living to witness their middle daughter's dramas. After all, my two siblings and I felt we were raised to maintain certain standards in life, being the best in all ways possible. A year went by while my husband vacillated about signing the divorce papers; I lived in a townhome with my youngest daughter who was graduating from high school and took a job with a small company which erected parking garages. Nine months later, and coping with daily migraines, I was told that the company was cutting back on expenses, and because I was the new employee, they had to let me go.

This was a true blessing and turning point in my life. My youngest daughter graduated from high school, I moved to California with a new business partner and then, into my forties, I launched the second phase of my work experience. I began to sense a higher purpose. Carolyn Myss calls this the "career" stage of our lives. The career of importing natural health products for an Australian company catapulted me into new realms of experience and self-confidence. My interest and research in natural health for many years helped to prepare me for this new venture. My children were grown and no longer living at home, which afforded me time to fully concentrate on my business. The next four years were an exciting and fulfilling time. The business prospered but came to a screeching halt when the Australian company decided to move their offices to the states and offer us a smaller position which we sensed would not last. We felt devastated. For several months the attorneys bickered and walked away with more money in their pockets than we did. Starting over again was an agonizing thought—how and where? Neither my partner nor I had saved much money as it was put back into our business venture.

A year later, through innumerable tears, anguish, and prayers, another opportunity opened for me, and at age forty-six I found myself stepping through the doorway which Carolyn Myss calls your third stage: your "vocation." I decided to begin writing a book on Australian tea tree oil, an Australian herb. In 1990, my new book publishing venture began and through the period of the next twelve years I wrote and published more books and helped a few other authors do the same. Much of my direction came from reading voluminous amounts of publishing material, attending workshops. and using my sixth sense. I felt for the first time a real sense of purpose, enthusiasm, and fulfillment. There were a few unfortunate experiences along my path, however. One of my authors absconded with twenty cases of books out of my office while I was away on Christmas holiday. She had been under contract granting her the rights to buy her books for her own marketing. She never responded to any of my calls for payment. Hiring an attorney was economically unfeasible for me at the time. I contacted a publishing remaining company in New York City (a remaining company purchases books from publishing houses at a deep discount and sells them at a cost below the original retail). We agreed upon a price they would pay my company and the rest of the stock of the books was shipped east.

Another difficult lesson came from a children's book project. This project contained stories and beautiful photographs of impoverished children around the world. It was a giant step from my traditional genre of natural healing, but I became enthralled with the idea and the financial opportunities it could afford me. The book would be presented on national television with the possibility of the celebrated Oprah Winfrey producing and narrating a television special. Of course, my head was swirling with endless possibilities. The author and I agreed to a contract, and she whisked off to Europe for a book symposium with marketing material in hand, which my business provided.

The floor collapsed upon her return. She informed me that she was going to cancel the contract and take it to another publishing house. She even told the woman photographer whose images she was using for the book that she found another photographer. As it happened, she met a male photographer at the conference, fell madly in love with him, and was going to have him take over the photographic project. The entire episode lasted a few months, causing me much humiliation and distress, but I had to move on. In retrospect, I realized I had allowed my ambition and success to get in the way of sound reasoning.

Ponzi Scheme

During the time in which my business was going through the challenges I mentioned, a friend approached me about an investment group that was paying back dividends up to 20 percent. She had received a great amount from her original investment. I was unaware of Ponzi schemes at the time, and I trusted her. Here again, greed and perhaps desperation played a part in my decision to invest some savings into the investment group. I do recall when writing the check that things did not feel right, but I mailed the money anyway. Shortly after that, the Ponzi scheme came to a screeching halt. I never received a dime back. I discovered afterward that people like my friend were being paid dividends from the latest investors' money and when the time was ripe the schemers shut the business down and hid the money, leaving the investors at a total monetary loss. A class action suit was brought, but because there were many people in the investment group throughout the US, very little money was recovered to be dispersed among the group. I spoke to an artist from Manhattan who had lost over $200,000. One of the men behind the Ponzi scheme was a medical doctor with disabilities. He was indicted along with some other people. Although these experiences were painful at the time, I learned a great deal more about myself during those trying times. Resiliency and optimism played a positive part in my emotional recovery. And I found I was able to forgive myself and others in order for me to continue down the path.

The vocation stage in my life has represented the culmination of years of work achievements and experiences which now give rise to a higher purpose. For instance, I had been drawn to natural health for over thirty years. That interest propelled me through various jobs as a health food manager, product importer, researcher, health writer, author, and publisher. I believe we all have unique callings during our lifetimes. I have immense gratitude for teachers and even the heartache experiences that have crossed my path throughout these years. What is your calling?

The whole purpose of education is first to prepare you with essential knowledge for the next stage in your life and then to persuade, coerce and convince you to use that knowledge in the hope that you will not, because of ignorance, be a destructive force to yourself and to others. Of course, you will forget details and facts, but all these years of learning in the areas of human knowledge will compel you nevertheless to remember at least where essential knowledge is to be found, or even re-discovered when you need it.

—Pearl Buck

Grown Children: Their Family and Finances

My grown children struggle more than I did during my formative years. They are faced with a climate of challenging economic times while they raise their children, have jobs, and find valued time to spend with themselves and their husbands. They have told each other that they didn't learn about finances from their parents while growing up; they had to learn this for themselves. From my perspective, we had them work during the summers, we gave them an allowance, and we tried to be sensible toward how money was spent. Looking back, I think more could have been done to demonstrate and teach them about finances and managing money. My husbands were both spendthrifts, which didn't help matters either. I found myself taking over the role of budgeting and paying the monthly bills. Finances and raising a family were still a challenge on many levels.

My eldest granddaughter graduated from a Colorado college. Two of my children did as well. Now I have other grandchildren attending higher education with more to follow. She told me that she has learned the value of money by having jobs throughout her four-year education. Her father has employed her and his son during school holidays and summer in his business. This is positive training for the working world which awaits them. Changes and challenges are to be expected in our lifetime. How we choose to deal with new opportunities and move forward is testament to our true selves. Can we live each day with positive and realistic attitudes, or will we dive into a cavernous hole of despair and fear?

Barn's burned down—now I can see the moon.

—Masahide (1657-1732),
Translated by Lucien Stryk

The Baby Boomer Generation Grows Up

As of 2023, over seventy-six million baby boomers born between 1946 and 1964 decreased to a population of roughly sixty-five million still surviving. While boomers may want to be young, they know they are getting older and need to plan accordingly. However, only 15 percent of boomers believe they are saving enough money to cover their future needs. Many boomers do not look forward to a leisurely retirement. The 2022 data for retirees aged sixty-four to sixty-five revealed that 80 percent of retirees believe they have enough money to live comfortably in retirement. The key goals included saving for unexpected emergencies and future medical problems, as well as saving for major purchases and fun activities, such as vacations. Our society tends to be very good at procrastination, and as a result, many boomers will find themselves, by necessity, working at a post-retirement age. The life expectancy of a healthy adult at age sixty-five is eighty years. There is a good chance that one of the spouses in a marriage will live beyond that, perhaps to ninety or more. The greatest risk is that they'll outlive their money.

The rule of thumb is to project post-retirement income at 75 percent of pre-retirement income. For example, if a couple earns $100,000 pre-retirement, $75,000 should meet their needs in retirement. The question is then, "What level of assets would support a $75,000 income?"

Based on a Monte Carlo Simulation (a technique that uses random numbers and probability to solve problems), the amount of available assets should be approximately $1.5 million to $2 million in order to provide an income of $75,000 per year. Let me explain further.

The Monte Carlo Simulation gives a framework that tells us how long our money will last given the rate of return on the money compared to the amount and rate of withdrawal. In simple terms, if you withdraw a higher percent than you are earning, at some point you will run out of money. Over the last 100 years the Standard and Poor's Index has averaged about a 10 percent return on investment. The index consists of 100 percent of large capitalization stocks which represent the largest portion of the economy—i.e., IBM®, Coca-Cola®, Microsoft®, Proctor and Gamble®, etc.

The average retiree should not hold all assets in stocks, but should have a balanced combination of stocks, fixed income investments (bonds, CDs, etc.), and a certain percentage in cash in a savings account or money market fund. Typically, an average retiree should have the following asset allocation: 50 to 60 percent in stocks, 30 to 35 percent in fixed income and the balance in savings.

As a result of this allocation, projected future returns could potentially be in the range of 7 to 8 percent. Going back to the assets available to generate these returns, as a rule of thumb, you could withdraw 4 to 5 percent of the return. The balance of the return should be reinvested in order to grow the assets to keep pace with inflation.

Simply put, if your portfolio is earning a total return of 8 percent and you are withdrawing 5 percent, there is a 3 percent surplus which is reinvested back into your portfolio, allowing the assets to grow. Remember, one of the spouses may live far beyond the average life expectancy, and as a result you not only need to preserve your assets but grow them.

The information in the section on baby boomer economics was contributed by my brother, Robert Baldanza. Robert was a financial adviser with a major brokerage firm and had been in the financial services business since 1970. He is now retired and lives in Florida with his wife of fifty-five years. They also have raised their grandson who was born with Cerebral Palsy who is now nineteen and thriving in school and in life.

Inheritance

According to a recent study of the Federal Reserve Board's Survey of Consumer Finances by the American Association of Retired People, about 85 percent of boomers expect to inherit nothing. A whopping 92 percent of the general population will receive no inheritance—4 percent will receive $25,000 or less; and only 1 percent of the population can expect to receive over $100,000 with the remaining two-fifths receiving between $25,000 and $100,000. It's becoming increasingly obvious that we cannot rely on family money, and the worldwide economic picture has put a stress on retirement accounts, company pensions, and investments to secure our future.

About ten years ago, I took a finance course from a woman whose father had a well-known US company that helped people prepare and file their yearly taxes. Her father was a professional icon in his field and yet when she had questions surrounding money she was told not to be concerned. As a result, she didn't comprehend how to manage her own assets until two husbands spent much of her wealth. It was at this point in her life she made the decision to learn everything she could about finances, wrote a book about her experience, and began to lecture and hold seminars for women around the country. We can continue to educate ourselves on how to manage and be smart with our money. There are many resources available on the internet, books, and financial courses.

Simplify

One way to manage our money is to simplify our lives. A local Denver news show told of an elderly woman who had lived on her property near train tracks and enjoyed the sounds of the trains going by only to have her home destroyed by a fire which was caused by sparks from a passing train. A couple of years before, she had turned down an offer of $1 million from a real estate developer. She said that she had no desire to sell. This was her home and she planned on staying there for the remainder of her life. All her possessions had been lost in the fire. What drew my attention was when asked by a reporter how she was coping in losing everything she responded, "You never see a person in Heaven with a U-Haul."

How can we choose to be more at peace in today's complex and anxious world? I made the decision to scale down financially and incorporate living more simply. While the cost of living has risen, I have had to learn to become a more conscious consumer.

Keys to Simplify

- Charge on a credit card only what can be paid off each month.
- Budget monthly money carefully.
- Buy clothes and household items at thrift and secondhand stores.
- Sell personal items on eBay® and Craigslist®.
- Consign expensive jewelry and antiques to help put more money into savings.

- Clean out closets every few months and either consign the contents or donate to a local thrift store.
- Household items not salable can go to organizations like Habitat for Humanity®.
- Shop for food more often, buying smaller quantities of produce that will be used in a few days.
- Look for items on the grocery shelf that are discounted.
- During the summer months, frequent local farmers' markets.
- Recycle and conserve on energy by biking rather than driving your car everywhere.
- Use more blankets on your bed during the colder months while lowering the thermostat.
- During the summer months plant a garden to provide some fresh vegetables, herbs, and fruit.
- In the warmer months have your family and friends enjoy the splendor of a summer evening with a picnic while listening to free music concerts.

Do not make despair your focus; rather have hope, gratitude, and love for the blessings you receive each day. Use these times to change things in your life that no longer serve. Simplify, reach out to family and friends and know that a positive attitude will bring you a brighter tomorrow.

Consider Relocating

I have lived from the East Coast of the US to the Hawaiian Islands. Some of the moves were related to job opportunities while others I found geographically appealing. My parents, grandparents, aunts, uncles, and siblings didn't move around. I was the adventurer and the nomad. I have kidded my brother and his family that if they ever decide to move out of the home, they have lived in for over forty years, it may take them another thirty to sort through all of their worldly possessions. When we move around, we don't have the time or ability to accumulate a lot of stuff. Living in various places has made me appreciate meeting new people and making friends along the way. The scenery changes and it opens up new doors for me to walk through.

I have hiked the Olympic Peninsula in the Northwest, seen eagles' nest, taken ferries to Canada, and kayaked along the shores. In Hawaii I swam in the warm Pacific waters, kayaked alongside the dolphins, and watched the whale's breach. I have shopped at outside farmers' markets, picked tropical flowers for my home and listened to the beautiful Hawaiian music. In Colorado, I ski with my family, plant my vegetable garden, have lawn picnics at summer music concerts, watch the first snowfall of the winter, sit by a beautiful river and bike and hike the trails. Perhaps none of these experiences would have happened for me if I had chosen to live in one place. Moving around is not for everyone, but for me it has been enchanting, exhilarating, and liberating. The idea of relocating is a lifestyle choice for many. The factors may be based on economics, health, or simply the desire to live elsewhere.

Population Growth and Demographics

As I was completing this section of the book, news agencies announced that the US population was officially at over 334 million people. The US population hit 200 million in 1967 and has grown 50 percent since that time, while production of goods and services accelerated by 217 percent. In thirty-five years, our population is projected to be 400 million, including (legal) immigrants. Baby boomers will be replaced with younger taxpayers, and the increased population will hopefully keep our economy thriving.

Even with the projected increase, the US will still have only one-sixth the population density of Germany, for instance, whose population is expected to stop growing within a few years. As of 2023, the world population is over 8 billion people. World population growth is 1.09 percent. The UN predicts that by 2050, the world population will be 9.15 billion people. The world's largest ethnic group is Han Chinese.

This information comes from wikipedia.com.

Population Distribution

Region	*Number*	*Percentage*
Asia	4,751,819,588	59.22%
Africa	1,460,476,458	18.2%
Europe	741,869,197	9.25%
North America	604,155,369	7.53%
South America	439,719,009	5.45%
Oceania	26,343,327	0.33%
Antarctica	4,000	0.02%
Total	**8,024,386,948**	**100.0%**

Some US states are also experiencing a decrease in population. Currently North Dakota, Ohio, Kansas, Maine, West Virginia, and Nebraska average fewer than fourteen households per square mile. A decrease in population will have an effect on the economy of those states and nations, as they must depend on younger generations to fill the economic gap.

More people now work remotely. which enables them to move around to other locations. Idaho, Utah, Montana and Florida have seen an increase in population. Taxes are higher in Illinois, New Jersey, New Hampshire, Connecticut and California. the higher cost of living exists in Hawaii, New York state, Connecticut and New Jersey.

According to The Center for Environment and Population, a nonpartisan research group in New Canaan, Connecticut, more than half the population of this country currently lives within fifty miles of the coasts. In a decade, with an additional twenty-five million people, half the total population increase will also be residing near the coasts. Along with this projected increase in population over the next decade, there will be an emergence of megacities, and twenty-five million more people will be seeking employment.

What impact this density will have on the environment is yet to be seen. Fragile water supplies in the desert areas of the Southwest may be affected, and low-lying areas of the southern states may be prone to hurricanes and massive flooding such as that experienced with Hurricane Katrina in 2005. States such as Colorado, Montana, and Northern California may experience diminished water supplies in their rivers. Personally, I have witnessed a population explosion in the last twenty years along the Colorado western slope, especially in the resort towns where more affluent people are seeking land and mountain properties.

We are also experiencing an increase in the number of Hispanics throughout the country. Expensive housing and costly real estate may drive less affluent people inland in the future. Tennessee's Hispanic population, for instance, is up 140 percent. By midcentury, when my grandchildren are between the ages of forty-four and sixty-two, the 34 percent population increase in the United States will have affected demographics, the environment, jobs, water supplies, energy distribution, and every other aspect of life, including retirement options.

Various regions within America indicate various personalities according to an extensive study done by Cambridge University. Extroverts are found more often in the Southeast, Midwest, and Great Plains states. Creative and open-minded people are living in the Northeast and on the West Coast. Fewer emotionally stable people may reside from Maine to Louisiana. Conscientious people tend to live in the South or Midwest. People may have a tendency to move to areas where they feel more comfortable, where they will fit in. Some may value the newness of an area in which they can reshape their thinking and develop new ideas of living and incorporate that into their health, occupations, and academic world.

Where Do You Want to Live?

Based on a survey of 450,000 adults, Colorado, New Mexico, and Hawaii capture three of the ten top spots where Americans can expect to live longest. How fortunate for me that I live in Colorado and can go to warmer climates during the winter months. There are currently over 500 centenarians in Colorado who have several surprising things in common regarding their lifestyles. They enjoy exercise and lots of sunshine (which all three of these states get plenty of); their diets are low in carbohydrates (which means more protein); they enjoy two to three ounces of alcohol intake per day, take multivitamins, and most have better-than-average educations. There are small cities and towns that are rated each year in the American Association of Retired Persons Livability Index. You can access all that information by going to their website. Check the Resource section at end of this book.

Elder Hostels

In 1975, Marty Knowlton was the co-founder of this international educational organization. He passed away in 2009 at age 88, leaving behind an incredible legacy. Elder hostels can be found in the fifty US states and over ninety countries. The not-for-profit provides over 8,000 educational programs in which over 160,000 people fifty-five years and older have participated. Ideas are exchanged through lectures, field trips, and travels. Many participate in hiking, photography, opera, birding, and water sports.

Living Outside of the US: Retirement Advantages

- Lower cost of living
- Real estate less expensive

- Lower taxes
- Cultural and recreational activities
- Quality of health care
- Telecommunications

South of the Border—Down Mexico Way

This song is being sung by US seniors heading south to capture less expensive housing and for their increasing health-care requirements. Living in another country may be daunting for some, but the idea of a mountain lake region brimming over with 40,000 to 80,000 American and European expatriates, along with a mild climate, is appealing to many.

- Nursing care costs in Mexico are much more affordable than in the US, making this move very appealing to baby boomers.
- There are only 288 nursing care facilities in Mexico, compared to over 9,000 in the US.
- The average cost for a private room in a Mexican nursing facility runs $18 to $50 per day compared to the US price of $206 (based on a 2006 MetLife insurance figure).
- In the United States, long-term care runs $2,500-7,000 per month compared to Mexico's $1,000-1,700 a month.
- One can also live in a studio apartment for $550/month which provides three meals a day, laundry, and cleaning services, and twenty-four-hour nursing care.
- Cost of living is extremely appealing, and the Mexican Social Security Institute (IMSS) provides full medical coverage to Americans for clinic and hospital costs. Medical coverage costs about $140 per year.

There are downsides to living in Mexico, however, with little or lax government regulations:

- Drug cartels have created an unsafe criminal environment in certain areas.
- Some nursing facilities suddenly go bankrupt, forcing people to find another place to live.
- Not all of the nursing facilities are class A.
- The Mexican government doesn't have strict codes, so many of the facilities are not monitored and two out of eight do not have State Health Department licenses.
- Medicaid, Medicare, Department of Veterans Affairs, and many US insurance companies will not cover any medical costs if you live in Mexico; to receive benefits from these US governmental organizations, you would have to return to the US for your medical care.

As more retirement and nursing communities crop up in places like Lake Chapala, Ensenada, Rosarita, Puerto Vallarta, Monterrey, and San Miguel de Allende, other homes have been forced to close due to poor management or unsanitary conditions. There is a bright future for increased and improved home-care facilities in Mexico. At the University of Texas in Austin, a forum made up of hospital administrators, insurance developers and policymakers convened to discuss the future of health-care facilities in Mexico. Tijuana's economic development council is asking the Mexican government to provide more federal funding to build more retirement facilities in Mexico. So, if "south of the border," Mexican cuisine, low-cost health care, and affordable living are calling you, check it out. You may just discover a new life.

Other Countries to Consider

- Panama
- Belize

- Costa Rica
- Ecuador
- Central America
- Argentina
- Thailand
- Greece
- Portugal

Important Considerations

- Cost of living
- Health care
- Country national health-care system
- Hospital care
- Safety and crime rates
- Taxes
- Paying US taxes
- Paying foreign taxes
- Senior benefits
- Collecting Social Security
- Banking
- Visas
- Immigration details
- Residency requirements
- Buying real estate

Seventy percent of people fifty and older choose to stay in their homes. Households that are sixty-five and older are expected to increase from 34 million to 48 million in the next two decades.

This information comes from Urban Institute.

Those who relocate seem more satisfied with change when they are seeking a more affordable cost of living, less pollution, and new friends.

Twenty-nine percent said they plan to relocate to another community. Respondents said they value communities that provide access to clean water, healthy foods, quality health care, and safe outdoor spaces.

Florida was the most popular destination, followed by North Carolina, Michigan, Arizona, and Georgia.

About 1 in 8 retirees who relocated out of state reported doing so to cut housing expenses, up from 1 in 15 in 2019. About 250,000 people relocated to other states in 2022.

Those who do move usually seek a warmer climate or move to be closer to family. Then there are those who never move (19 percent) and those who simply like their home and want to stay (14 percent). Those who relocate seem more satisfied with change when they are seeking a more affordable cost of living, less pollution, and new friends.

No matter where retirees reside and how they choose to live, we find that many “elders” of our society contribute their years of wisdom in their communities in a myriad of worthwhile ways.

For me, moving has been a way of life, although I have stayed "put' for thirteen years now. I live in snowy Colorado and do escape to visit Floridian family. I shall see what may lie ahead for me regarding a life in a more temperate zone.

We have every reason to look forward into the future with hope and excitement. Fear nothing and no one. Work honestly. Be good, be happy. And remember that each of you is unique, your soul your own, irreplaceable, and individual in the miracle of your mortal frame.

—Pearl Buck

Boomers Health-Care Challenges

Boomers want to be fit and healthy, and they are increasingly taking small steps to improve their well-being, primarily by eating healthy. But they still remain the most overweight age group in our nation. The latest data reveal that they find it tough to cut down on the bad stuff (e.g., alcohol and tobacco) and they exercise less.

Based on these habits, it is likely boomers will continue to be heavily dependent on health care, the escalating cost of which is their leading source of stress. But, in large part because of a likely sharp increase in health-care costs, the growth in consumption of medical products and services may be about to slow. With health-care accounting for only about 5 percent of boomers' expenditures, many employers believe there is still plenty of room for households to pay more for medical coverage. The catalyst for employees paying more could well be the Medicare Prescription Drug, Improvement and Modernization Act of 2003, which went beyond assisting seniors with prescription drugs and contained many other provisions that have wide-ranging implications for the entire health industry. A key provision of the act is the establishment of health savings accounts (HSAs) which will likely have profound implications for both employees and retirees. In effect, an HSA is to health care what a 401(k) is to retirement savings.

Hospice

Hospice is truly an incredibly caring organization. When they came into my brother's home during our sister's last days, they supported us each day with a gentle and compassionate approach. They were there for less than a week and having them there during the late-night hours helped us to step away for a short time and renew ourselves. After Pat died, the staff said how our team effort was inspirational to them. They shared that so many families are discomfited and ill at ease at the experience of seeing a loved one preparing to die. They leave it up to the Hospice team to handle everything. Our mutual desire was to be totally present for our sister. We played music and talked to her, even though toward the end she wasn't able to communicate. She was adamant regarding staying with us rather than being admitted to a hospital. Our loving efforts, and those of the Hospice workers, hopefully made her last days easier.

One out of three Americans call upon Hospice when a member of their family may have six months or less to live. There are organizations around the world. Hospice provides comfort in a home setting for the terminally ill. A support team may include a physician, a nurse, a home health aide, a social worker, a chaplain, and a volunteer. One can contact Hospice for an international directory of Hospice organizations.

Right to Die

I am grateful that none of my family members has suffered a coma or has been hooked up to life support systems for long periods of time. They had the finances to live in their homes, have live-in help, and pay doctor and hospital bills. I read once that dying in one's sleep used to be more the norm and the best and most natural way to die. My grandmother Jennie passed in her sleep. Morality, religion, and laws support the stance that euthanasia should be treated as a crime. At this time there are nine states that permit a right to die provision: California, Washington, Colorado, District of Columbia, Hawaii, Maine, New Jersey, Vermont, and Oregon. The World Federation of Right to Die Societies supports a person deciding when he or she wishes to die. Belgium, Netherlands, Switzerland, and Luxembourg all support a final exit network. Many countries support people.

This information comes from www.wfrtds.org.

Death is nothing at all. It does not count. I have only slipped away into the next room. Nothing has happened. Everything remains exactly as it was. I am I, and you are you, and the old life that we lived so fondly together is untouched, unchanged. Whatever we were to each other, that we are still. Call me by the old familiar name. Speak of me in the easy way, which you always used. Put no difference into your tone. Wear no forced air of solemnity or sorrow. Laugh as we always laughed at the little jokes that we enjoyed together. Play, smile, think of me, and pray for me. Let my name be ever the household word that it always was. Let it be spoken without an effort, without the ghost of a shadow upon it. Life means all that it ever meant. It is the same as it ever was. There is absolute and unbroken continuity. What is death but a negligible accident? Why should I be out of mind because I am out of sight? I am but waiting for you, for an interval, somewhere very near, just around the corner. All is well.

—Henry Scott Holland

Tooth Care Truth in the USA

An estimated 77 million Americans do not carry dental insurance. Having regular checkups and maintaining healthy teeth and gums not only saves our teeth but helps to ward off certain diseases of the body including heart disease.

There Are Insurance Options for Dental Insurance Although They Don't Cover All Dental Procedures.

- The American Association of Retired Persons offers dental insurance through Delta Dental which operates like an HMO. In other words, they provide a national list of dentists under their plan, and you must use one of these dentists to be covered.

- Care Credit is a charge card to be used for dental procedures; one needs to use a dentist on their list and apply for a certain amount of credit; they provide an interest free period after which there is a high interest fee applied on the remaining balance.
- In order to cut costs, some people go to a local dental college where supervised students do the work at considerably lower cost.
- Some go to Mexico for treatment.
- Caring Hands (caringhandsworldwide.org)

If any of these ideas are not an option for you, it would be wise to research different policies, especially if you are self-employed or if your employer doesn't provide dental insurance.

Organizations that provide dental and medical relief include Worldwide Dental Relief and Global Dental Relief (globaldentalrelief.org) These organizations provide free dental and medical care to thousands of impoverished people around the globe.

Shopping for Pharmaceuticals

Twenty thousand prescription drugs have been approved through the FDA and 66% of adults take prescription drugs in America.

Opioids kill over 50,000 people per year, while tranquilizers, prescription stimulants, and benzodiazepines are the most commonly abused drugs.

The single biggest factor is that drug manufacturers operating out of the U.S. and wholesalers cannot set drug prices as they'd like. There are fewer intermediaries or go-betweens in the Canadian pharmaceutical chain who often mark up prices as there are in the United States of America.

The FDA allows customers to purchase drugs from Canadian online pharmacies and have them shipped to the U.S. under the same guidelines that regulate bringing drugs across the border. That means that you will need a valid prescription from a licensed health care provider and the drugs must be approved for use in the U.S.

The U.S., Chile, Switzerland, and Mexico have the highest prescription drug prices.

In recent years, Americans—many of them older—have spent between $500 million and $1 billion annually on prescription medicines coming from Canada, where brand-name drugs, including those made by US companies, are often much cheaper than the same medication purchased in the US Although cross-border shipments of medications have been illegal for some time, authorities did little to stop the practice until late in 2004. At that time, the Department of Homeland Security began a crackdown on drugs being shipped into this country from Canada. By November 2005, the Department of Homeland Security's customs and border protection had seized over 39,000 packages of Canadian drugs coming into the United States. Recently, due largely to the hue and cry from retirees and various congressmen and women, DHS has backed off this policy somewhat.

However, before ordering prescription drugs from Canada or elsewhere, it would be wise to check the law and current enforcement policy. Refer to the resource section at the back of the book.

What America's Health Care Could Learn from Five Other Countries

The United States has been rated thirty-seventh in the world for fairness and quality of health care by the WHO. We are a nation regulated by the pharmaceutical and medical industries. Until we have a leader of this country who doesn't have deep involvement with the special interest groups that support those institutions, we as seniors will continue to be at the mercy of accelerated medical costs and limited health-care options, which I strongly believe should include preventive medicine like acupuncture, Chinese medicine, chiropractors, and massage therapists. This also includes professionals who are interested in teaching people how to have healthier lifestyles through preventive measures and thus eliminating many diseases which older people are susceptible to.

Health Care Around Our World

I watched a Public Broadcasting Program, *Sick Around the World* which discusses other countries' health-care reforms. This program is educational and informative, although certainly not perfect. Perhaps the US can learn lessons from other parts of the world and incorporate progressive changes in our especially flawed health-care system.

United Kingdom

The British are high on complementary medicine and herbs. If it's good enough for the Queen and her family, it must be great for the common people too. The Brits pay for their health-care coverage through taxes which still equates to one-half of what Americans pay.

- The government owns the hospitals.
- Doctors are government employees.
- No insurance or medical bills.
- No medical bankruptcy.
- The wait for emergency primary care heart and hip surgeries is less than six months.
- Patients have a choice which hospital they can go to.
- Patients receive incentives to stay healthy.

Japan

They are the second richest country in the world with a population of 130 million people. All Japanese are covered under a one payment system. Insurance companies are not allowed to make a profit. The downside is that 50 percent of Japanese hospitals experience financial difficulties.

- Highest life expectancy in the world.
- Lowest infant mortality.
- Government pays for the poor.
- Eight percent of hospitals and physicians are private.
- People can see any specialist of their choice.
- No appointments necessary and may go often.
- Longer hospital stays.
- Twice the amount of hospital scans performed per capita compared to the US and Britain.
- Medical prices for procedures and drugs re-negotiated every two years.
- MRI cost is $98 compared to $2,500 in the US.
- Hospital stays cost $10 per day, $90 for a private room. (In Japan, a private room can contain up to four people.)
- Medical machines are inexpensive to manufacture and are exported worldwide.
- Doctors cannot get rich.
- If a Japanese citizen loses his job, they do not lose their insurance.
- Employees pay half of the $280/month family health

premium.

Some New Health-Care Options

You may be able to cut medical costs by going to a local medical school or finding a nurse practitioner. You might also want to explore TeleDoc (800-835-2362), which offers consultations by telephone. The initial registration fees are small, and there is a small monthly fee for these services. There are over 200 TeleDoc physicians listed in this network. Also, some retail stores and pharmacies have opened in-house clinics with a reasonable ($25 to $60) fee for an appointment.

Germany

In 1880 Chancellor Otto von Bismarck established health-care reform which was named the Bismarck Plan. Germany is now the third richest country in the world. Germany has private doctors and hospitals. Medical school is free although physicians do not receive high salaries compared to doctors in the US. With over 240 private insurance providers available, they can compete for business but are not allowed to make a profit. Hospitals are not allowed to raise their prices. The government renegotiates hospital charges every year.

- All German people are offered health care.
- The wealthy can elect to opt out and pay privately.
- Ninety percent of Germans are insured.
- Health care includes medical, dental, optical, and counseling.
- Homeopathy and spa treatments included.
- Short wait for doctor appointments.
- People pay health premiums based on their personal incomes.

- Workers can split their premiums with their employers 50 percent.
- If they lose their job, they do not lose their insurance coverage.
- Pregnant women receive free health care.

Switzerland

Switzerland reformed their health-care program in 1994. In this country of over 8 million, there is no medical bankruptcy. (US has as many as 700,000 per year).

- The country pays for the poor.
- Everyone is offered health insurance coverage, and no one is turned down.
- Pharmaceutical companies rated in the top ten in the world.
- Administrative costs are 5.5 percent compared to the US, which can range between 20 to 30 percent.
- Monthly family premiums cost $750.
- Uninsured are required to pay their own medical bills.

Taiwan

This island contains twenty-three million people and is considered wealthy. A health-care program was initiated in 1995 by comparing the best health programs selected from ten to fifteen developed countries and choosing the best from each to incorporate into the Taiwan health reform. There is no medical bankruptcy, although the system is under strain due to rising medical costs.

- Free choice of doctors and no wait time for appointments.
- All medical expenses are covered, including traditional Chinese medicine.
- National insurance system with one government provider.

- Administrative costs are less than 2 percent per year.
- Smart card assigned to each person with their health history recorded into a national system.

Mixing foreign travel for pleasure, while seeking lower cost medical services, seems to be growing in popularity. Many foreign hospitals have US-trained physicians, and their rates are easily half that of similar care in the US, especially for orthopedics, dentistry, and plastic surgery. Some of the most popular countries providing lower cost medical services are India, Africa, Thailand, and Costa Rica. If you choose to explore these options, please check credentials carefully and, if possible, speak to someone who has been through the procedure you are seeking.

Step 7

Forget Your Age: Live Now!

The Best Way to Live Your Life

Some of us made our riches early in life and retired at a young age to less stressful living, where we have a multitude of life choices to pick from. Some of us are still working toward the day we can hang up our hat and hope to have a generous nest egg tucked away, a comfortable pension, and other investments to assist in living out the remainder of our years in relative comfort. Some of us take what we have and head to areas of the world where our money stretches farther, the cost of living is lower, and we can settle into a comfortable home surrounding ourselves with like-minded people. If we have time on our hands, we may even start an online business or take on other part-time endeavors.

Some of us, however, do not have the luxury to stop working. Our Social Security payments will not cover our monthly living expenses and we do not have enough savings to live off for the remainder of our lives; or we have too much debt to manage without a steady income. We feel we have no option other than to "play the hand that's been dealt."

Whichever position you find yourself in during this time of your life, there are always options to choose from. I have been single for over twenty-five years and have been self-employed most of my adult life. Thus, my Social Security benefits are slimmer, I am not entitled to a pension, and my savings are clearly not enough for me to stop working. As dismal as that may sound to some and familiar to others, I have many blessings in my life. I have my health, family, beautiful places where I have lived, great friends, and an everlasting presence of spiritual comfort, love, and inner peace to sustain me in the most challenging times. I still have an alert mind and healthy body to continue creating more abundance in my life.

Aging may bring about risks to the mind and body, such as memory loss, Alzheimer's or dementia, but ongoing research has found good reason to feel better about growing older.

According to Elkhonon Goldberg, professor of neurology at New York University School of Medicine, aging does not always lead to loss and deterioration; it can also bring about rebirth and renewal. Professor Goldberg is the author of *The Wisdom Paradox: How Your Mind Can Grow Stronger as Your Brain Grows Older*. It seems that neuroplasticity, the ability to develop new neurons, is stimulated in people who keep their minds continually active as they age.

Goldberg cites Albert Einstein as a prime example. "When he wasn't working, he played the violin to keep his mind sharp." Goldberg emphasizes the importance of continually challenging our brains by "stepping out of our comfort zone and our repetitive routines" (Goldberg, 2006). I now have a greater understanding of and appreciation for the long-term benefits of the board games, bridge, and other card games I played as a child and throughout my life.

My grandmother started walking five miles a day when she was sixty. Now she's ninety-seven years old and we don't know where the heck she is!

—Ellen Degeneres

Sexuality

The adage "use it or lose it" could be appropriate to many of us as we age. We may need to put more emphasis on creating sexual excitement. Our hormone production may have decreased but surely our desires to be held and satisfied are still hovering around us. True, it may take longer for us to become aroused, and we may need more time to reach orgasm, but it is worth it to include this special intimacy in our lives. Common knowledge is that, along with the normal changes of aging, sometimes health conditions and medications play a part for men in achieving an erection. Diabetes, depression, high blood pressure, and prostate problems can all play a role in diminished performance. Pre- and post-menopausal symptoms in women may decrease sexual desires. Addiction to liquor, cigarettes, or drugs certainly doesn't help, either. However, there are many natural herbal treatments available to help men and women increase their sexual desire and performance. Ask your health practitioner what he or she may recommend that wouldn't interfere with any medications you may be taking.

Healthy sexual activity has many benefits. Sex is great aerobic exercise—equivalent to walking up two flights of stairs. It can slow aging and perhaps make those eye wrinkles go away. The more sexual contact you have, the more your body will naturally produce more sex hormones which bolster immune systems and strengthen muscles and bones. There is a humorous true story about sex coming from a large (twelve-story!) German brothel that offers a 50 percent discount for seniors. The director, Armin Lobscheid, implied that all clients need to do is show some proof of age. He said that there's plenty of demand and people have certainly been taking advantage of the offer, and that older folks are more active than what people may think. This certainly sounds like more fun than senior movie or restaurant discounts.

If you don't have that special person to snuggle up next to, there is always a place in our hearts to express love to those close to us.

Sex is 50 percent of what you got, and 50 percent of what others think you got.

—Sophia Loren

Is Retirement for You?

By 2024, nearly one in four people in the labor force are projected to be age fifty-five or over. This is a big change from 1994, when people ages fifty-five and older represented only 11.9 percent of the labor force—a share smaller than those held by other age groups: sixteen to twenty-four, twenty-five to thirty-four, thirty-five to forty-four, and forty-five to fifty-four.

The labor force is expected to increase by 8.9 million, or 5.5 percent, from 2020 to 2030. The labor force of people ages sixteen to twenty-four is projected to shrink by 7.5 percent from 2020 to 2030. Among people ages seventy-five years and older, the labor force is expected to grow by 96.5 percent over the next decade.

This information comes from TED: The Economics Daily.

The pandemic has dramatically affected people working from offices. Worldwide, a higher percentage of people now work remotely.

By the end of 2023, 48 percent of knowledge workers globally will be working either hybrid or fully remotely—up from 27 percent in 2019, according to a January survey by management consultancy Gartner.

There has been a notable increase in the percentage of people remaining in the labor force in each age cohort from fifty-five and older. This increase in labor market engagement is likely due to several factors. These include the elimination of the mandatory retirement age in various provinces, the ability to defer Canadian Pension Plan (CPP) benefits, the increase in service sector jobs, and the fact that people are generally healthier today than prior generations of the same age. The high cost of living has created an older workforce because many people believe they will outlive their savings. (Orlando, 2023.)

Twenty years from now, you will be more disappointed by the things you did not do than the things you did do. So, throw off the bowlines. Sail away from the safe harbor. Catch the trade winds in your sails. Explore, dream, discover.

—Mark Twain

Keep Inspired

It seems highly appropriate to address not only the over-fifty crowd and the baby boomers in this book, but the older generation as well. Living in Hawaii, I have witnessed phenomenal strength, energy, endurance, and discipline during the world-famous Ironman Triathlon. I have seen people in their seventies and eighties complete this grueling test of courage; some even in wheelchairs. I have asked myself, "What drives them to do this?" Perhaps it gives them a purpose and keeps them in the game of life. We are not all athletes of that superior ability; however, we are athletes of a different sort. We thrive on challenge, we continue to learn, and most of all, we believe we can continue to create a full life into our sunset years.

My eighty-four-year-old maternal grandfather surrounded himself with young people. He read voraciously and spoke several languages. He owned several businesses and never officially retired. He believed by doing these things he was invigorated and stimulated by active dialogue and the exchange of ideas and ideals with others, younger and older alike.

I recently read an article about an athlete named Erwin Jaskulski, who held world records in track in the ninety-five to ninety-nine and one hundred plus age groups. He passed away in 2006 at the age of 103. Even at 101, he was studying his technique to see how he could improve. He became an inspiration to others through his example of commitment and discipline. Not only was he an athlete, but he also pursued interests in music, philosophy, and could hold a lively discussion on a variety of subjects. His main philosophy was "to be happy and joyful in life."

Gilad of the Hawaiian TV show, *Gilad's Bodies in Motion*, once saw Jaskulski on the beach doing some incredible feats of exercise, standing on his head, running, doing push-ups, and thought Jasulski was amazing for a man in his sixties—only to discover he was eighty-two at the time! He and Jaskulski developed a lasting friendship.

The Remarkable Story of Jack LaLanne

In January 2011, Jack LaLanne passed away from pneumonia at age ninety-six. Almost up to the end of his life, Jack continued to follow his passion for healthy living. Jack LaLanne's dad died at age fifty, but obviously Jack didn't believe genetics controlled longevity. He truly believed man could live to 150.

For more than a half century, the name Jack LaLanne had been synonymous with fitness, proper diet, and good health. He was often referred to as the "Godfather of Fitness." In 1934, at the age of twenty-one, he opened the first modern health spa in Oakland, California and continued on to introduce exercise to television in 1951 on the popular *Jack LaLanne Show*.

Jack LaLanne's life was transformed at age fifteen when he attended a lecture given by the health pioneer Paul Bragg. At the time, Jack was sickly, hooked on sugar, and had a "junk food" diet. From that moment he was changed forever.

Into his nineties, Jack continued to monitor his diet, exercise, and take supplements. His website sold his books and supplements, and before his death, he could be seen on television demonstrating and selling his juicer with the same trademark enthusiasm.

Jack's philosophy regarding healthy longevity consisted of the following:

- Exercise regularly and practice good nutrition.
- Have a plan.

- Too many people spend time watching television and drinking.
- Get your priorities straight.

"You have to work at longevity," he noted in an exclusive interview with Life Extension®. He believed that a sound program of physical fitness could lead to a productive and healthy life in our golden years. He recommended staying away from animal fats and processed foods and reading food labels: if you cannot understand the ingredients, don't buy it.

- He worked out from 5:00 a.m. to 7:00 a.m. each day.
- His meals were at 11:00 a.m. and 7:00 p.m.
- His morning meal consisted of four to eight egg whites and five pieces of fresh fruit, often prepared with his juicer.
- He and his wife ate out at restaurants that would prepare meals he requested; not all of us have this luxury, however, and can duplicate much of this in our own kitchens.
- He ate salads comprised of many vegetables, with fish and turkey for protein.
- He ate whole grains.
- He avoided red meat and dairy products.
- His supplements consisted of everything from A to Z, including fish oil, cod liver oil, all of the vitamins, minerals, and enzymes.

In his early years, Jack had to fight conventional medical wisdom which held that weightlifting would make athletes muscle-bound and inflexible, turn women into men, and put the elderly in an early grave. He was hopeful for the future because medical professionals now recognize the importance of daily exercise as part of a prescription for good health.

"Medical schools are now putting more emphasis on the value of nutrition and exercise, so future doctors can help people live longer," he noted. "Young doctors are now prescribing these things and the older ones are slowly realizing their importance. People need to change their patterns if they are going to increase their longevity. Even people in their eighties and nineties can benefit from exercise." Despite the considerable progress made in the last sixty years, LaLanne recognized that there was always room for improvement. "Even with all the scientific knowledge we have on the benefits of exercise, there are more fat people than ever," he noted with regret. "What we need is consumer education. People in the health field need to bind together to overcome the brainwashing that results from hawking junk food on TV" (Tuttle, 2006).

"We have to start with the educational system, to teach our youth the right way to lead their lives. Kids are creatures of habit, so you have to get them to do the right thing and forget all that negative advertising they see on television. Until that's done, we won't make real headway in our campaign" (Tuttle, 2006).

Up until his death at age ninety-six, Jack LaLanne remained the eternal optimist. He had seen so much improvement since he started his crusade that he remained idealistic about the eventual triumph of the fitness lifestyle over a sedentary existence with its television, video games, junk food, and early death. "Nutrition and exercise should be an important part of everyone's life," he said. "Life should be a happy adventure, and to be happy you need to be healthy. Just take things one step at a time and remember that everything you do takes energy to achieve. You need to plant the seeds and cultivate them well. Then you will reap the bountiful harvest of health and longevity" (Tuttle, 2006).

He laid the groundwork for others to have exercise programs, and now it has bloomed from that black and white program into a colorful enterprise.

—Former California Governor Arnold Schwarzenegger

Barbara Holden—Artist Extraordinaire

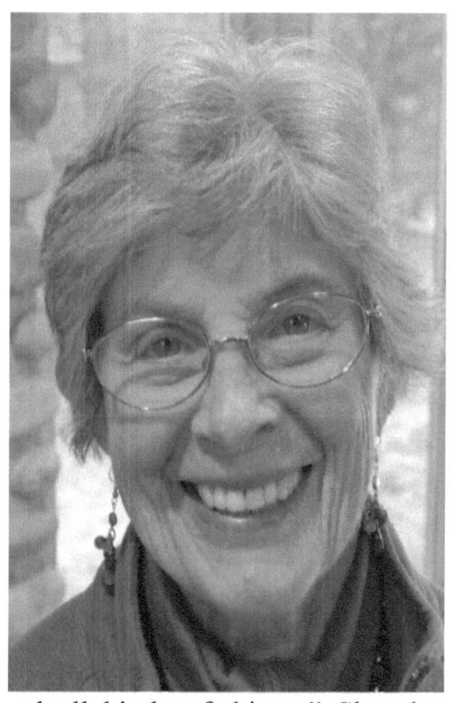

As my dear friend Barbara prepared for her ninety-first birthday, being treated for cancer has not slowed down. We met for walks although she wasn't her peppy self. Her attitude was still uplifting and her gratitude for all her life experiences remained positive. Barbara was a graduate of Vassar College in NY, graduating in 1951 with a major in social anthropology. Barbara said, "This also meant I majored in '105' courses—all those introductory courses on various subjects—because they were 'all culture.' I learned all kinds of things." She also minored in art. During her college years, she spent her summers working in Glacier National Park in Montana/Canada. After she married Stuart, who worked with the Ford Foundation, he took her to England where she started her family. They were relocated to India and Geneva, Switzerland. After returning stateside, Barbara went for her master's degree in art. Barbara attended the Cleveland Institute of Art to obtain her BA and MA. After periods of living and traveling in Germany, Holland, and Mexico, they finally settled back in the USA in two homes: Chatham, Cape Cod for six months and Vail, CO for six months. Stuart, a Scotsman, loved to be near the sea, and Barbara loved the mountains and skiing.

Barbara continued to pursue skiing, hikes, and created beautiful botanical art as well as teaching to a select small group of art students at her home. She was a member of the American Society of Botanical Artists and the Rocky Mountain Society of Botanical Artists. Twenty-four hours before she made the decision to end her life through the Colorado Right to Die, she was creating a new painting with her son.

Her mother had a nervous breakdown when she was young which gave her and her twin unsupervised time to have many adventures together. Barbara still displayed the sense of adventure in her daily life, which also included singing and playing her keyboard. Healthy food was perhaps Barbara's greatest passion. "I was brought up to believe one should eat morally, that you are what you eat. That's why my father moved us to the country, so we could raise our own food. We canned everything. And we never had many sweets in the house. And even today, since I'm not used to them, sweet things upset my stomach. When I was in college, kids made fun of me because I would eat so many fruits and vegetables. When we lived in India, the vegetarian cuisine was so good that I gave up eating meat."

On exercise, Barbara said, "Keeping the body fit is vitally important to me. Exercising is so important, especially as you age." Barbara was consistent with her daily exercises: stretching, walking, winter activities, and yoga classes. Barbara's mantra was that life needs laughter and fun for balance along life's journey. Barbara was a jewel and an inspiration. I foresee her marching on in the heavenly realms.

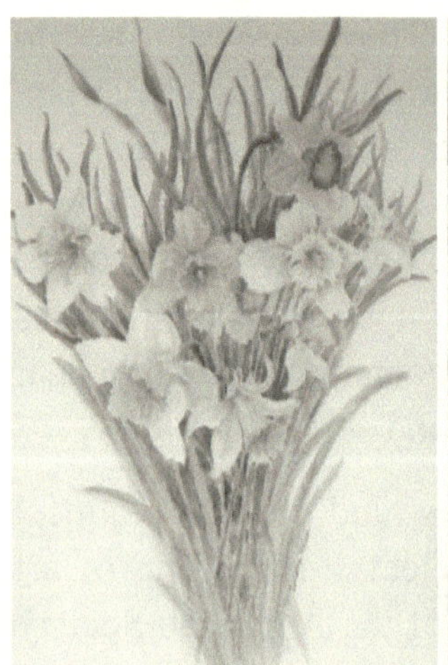

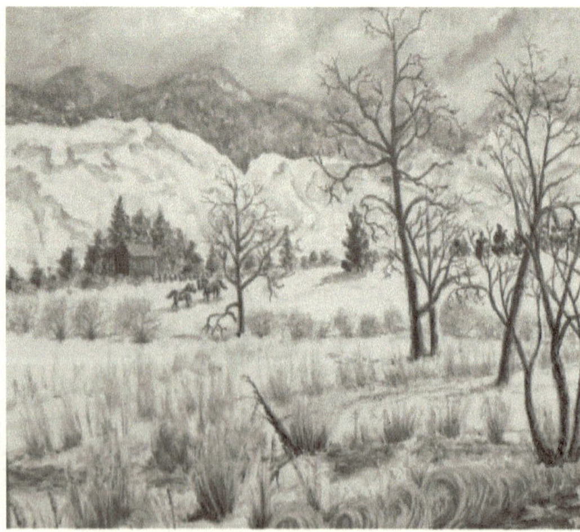

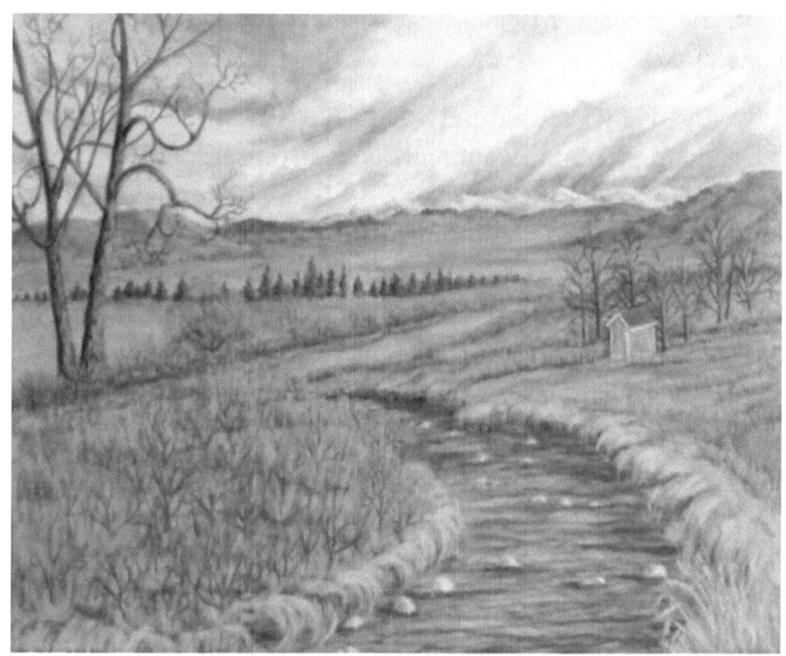

A Final Tribute

Barbara K. Holden, aged 91, passed away peacefully 9/25/21, with her children at her side following a battle with ovarian cancer.

Barbara grew up in rural Ohio with her identical twin sister, Connie, and her older sister, Janet. She had degrees from Vassar College and the Cleveland Institute of Art. She met and married Stuart Holden from Glasgow, Scotland, in 1951. They moved to Great Britain where they lived for seven years and had the first two of their three children, Steve and Sandy. Connie was born in Cleveland shortly after they returned from Great Britain. In 1961 they moved to live in India for three years. After that the family traveled widely and lived for extended periods in Spain, Switzerland, Germany, and Mexico. Barb had strong interests in art and music throughout her life. She sang in groups as a member or as a soloist and taught art in schools, art centers, and privately. She taught painting through the last week of her life. She was a painter, weaver, potter, and creator of multiple art forms. After studying Botanical Arts in the Field Study Centers in England, she joined the

American, Rocky Mountain and New England Societies of Botanical Art.

For twenty-five years, she and Stuart lived in Vail, CO in the winter and Chatham, MA in the summer. They loved the outdoors; in Vail, they were founding members of Vail Club 50 and lead the cross-country and snowshoeing groups for many years. Barb was active with PEO, singing in the Dicken's Carolers, the choir of the Presbyterian Church in Avon, and in local art groups. In Chatham, MA she was also a steward for Samuel Hawes Park and the Coastal Plains Ponds Habitat as a docent, photographer of animals and plants, and in clearing the ever-thriving poison ivy from the walking path. In 2014, four years after Stuart's death, Barb moved to Eagle, CO to live full time and immediately immersed herself in the volunteer and art world. She joined the Vail Valley Art Guild and had several art showings. She practiced yoga and played Mahjong. She loved walking and gardening in the summer and enjoyed snowshoeing and cross-country skiing in the winter.

Barb was an inspiration for eating wholesomely (no sugar!), eating frugally (an enormous breakfast followed by much smaller or non-existent meals later), and exercising diligently and faithfully every day. She was loved and respected and left a mark on this world that was so much bigger than her petite frame.

Longevity in Other Lands

The Okinawa Centenarian Study (OSG) is a twenty-five-year study based on solid evidence:

- People of Okinawa have a lower mortality and chronic disease rate compared to US, which ranks eighteenth.
- They are lean and fit, they are strong boned, with healthy hormone levels, and have low rates of dementia, cancer, and cardiovascular disease.
- Families care about their elders; they are not forgotten and shoved away in nursing homes until they die.

- Stress is virtually non-existent.
- Their diet consists of fish, vegetables, plenty of fresh water, and green tea.
- They practice tai chi, dance, walk, and garden, all natural and pleasurable forms of exercise.

Other areas where the people live longer, healthier lives are:

- Andora (France), Macau (near China), San Marion (Italy), Singapore, Hong Kong, Japan, Sweden, Switzerland, and Guernsey (near the English Channel).
- India is known to have the lowest level of Alzheimer's worldwide; the correlation may be their diet, which includes spices like turmeric which aids in anti-inflammatory responses in the body.

The One-Hundred-Year-Old Club

In the small Southern Italian village of Acciaroli and tiny communities nearby, age is just a number. There is an escape from dementia, heart disease, and other illnesses, which are prevalent in western society. Besides having a Mediterranean diet consisting of fruit, fish, vegetables, and olive oil, there has been a link to a hormone that widens blood vessels. Researchers at San Diego School of Medicine and at Sapienza University in Rome have stated Adrenomedullin is present in a much-reduced quantity in the subjects studied and seems to act as a powerful protecting factor, helping the optimal development of microcirculation, or capillary circulation. As people age, capillaries degenerate; however, this is not the case here. The older people's capillaries resemble those of twenty-year-olds. A San Diego cardiologist named Dr. Alan S. Maisel is performing blood tests along with cardiac and neurological tests. There are also factors being considered regarding genetics, lifestyle, diet, and physical activities. This is much like some of the other countries mentioned in this section.

They consume rosemary every day and walk, fish, and garden. Their sex lives are extremely active. They are Italians, after all!

France

I've already mentioned the Mediterranean diet and its health benefits regarding Alzheimer's. Now from France, land of wine, cheese, and rich sauces, there is another revelation in health and longevity. While Japan has the longest life expectancy at an average of over eighty-five and a half years, France averages eighty-four years, and increases three months a year. So, by the turn of this century, the average life span for French women will be ninety-five and men ninety-one years of age. Compare Americans' average life expectancy at just over eighty years.

In 2006, more than 16,000 French hit the centenarian mark; that number has doubled in the last seven years. According to the National Institute of Statistics and Economic Studies, there will be more than 150,000 centenarians in France by 2050. Longer life expectancy is spreading throughout Europe. Health care has improved along with lowered risks of drinking, smoking, and accidents. The people who live in the Southwest region of the Pyrenees in France may indulge in their local wines and rich foie gras from duck and goose liver yet live longer than their fellow citizens who reside in northern areas. French women live a more relaxed life, eat and drink in moderation, stay active, laugh a lot, and have a good time—an excellent example for all of us.

A French woman, Jeanne Calment, died in 1997 at the age of 122. She had the longest confirmed life span in the world. Not only did she live alone, but she took up fencing at age eighty-five, continued to ride her bike, and appeared in the movie *Vincent and Me* at age 114, making her the oldest actress in history. Jeanne met Vincent Van Gogh when she was fourteen, and found him to be "dirty, badly dressed, and disagreeable." She claimed that giving up smoking at the "youthful" age of 117 attributed to her longevity.

The One-Hundred-Year Mark

Centenarians, those who have reached the age of one hundred, currently number 50,454 in the United States alone. People who live 110 years, super centenarians, are estimated to number 450 worldwide. One in fifty women will live to be 100; for men, it is one in 200. Genetics play a strong factor, but also how people take care of themselves. A survey of healthy centenarians reveals that they credit their long life to their faith, a healthy diet, not smoking, and strong family bonds. To avoid crisis care, many place self-care and health care high in their priorities. Only 4 percent of this group fear death.

Eric Plasker, DC, author of *The 100 Year Lifestyle*, says that "being passionate about your life is the key to mastering your life" (Plasker, 2007). Look at the famous centenarian George Burns—smoking cigars nearly every day of his long life. I believe he must have been passionate about life; he certainly seemed to enjoy it to its fullest. L. Stephen Coles, MD, co-founder of the Gerontology Research Group, says that super centenarians escape from heart disease, cancer, and stroke. So, if we have made it that far, we must be doing something right.

The Old Wisdom

by Jane Goodall, retrieved from GoodReads.com.

When the night wind makes the pine trees creak
And the pale clouds glide across the dark sky,
Go out my child, go out and seek
Your soul: The Eternal I.

For all the grasses rustling at your feet
And every flaming star that glitters high
Above you, close up and meet
In you: The Eternal I.

Yes, my child, go out into the world; walk slow
And silent, comprehending all, and by and by
Your soul, the Universe, will know
Itself: the Eternal I.

Afterword

Afoot and light-hearted
I take to the open road
Healthy, free, the world before me
The long brown path Leading wherever I choose.

—*Walt Whitman*

The last several years since I left Hawaii have been a grand exploration that has required me to retrain my mind, release stress, worry less, and live in the present moment by "going with the flow."

Tragically, I lost two dear family members within the last three years; my eldest daughter, Tamara, as well as my nephew Nick. Tamara had uterine cancer. Nick through a drug overdose. I did my best to cope and grieve. I am not in control of others' destinies. I have beautiful memories of our times together. My daughter, who celebrated her fifty-fifth birthday with a small group of friends and family nine days before, had suffered so much that she was ready to depart this life. She left four grown children and six grandchildren. As they continue on their lives' journeys, they miss Mimi, as she was called. On occasion her favorite symbol the dragonfly, has appeared for us. At the age of thirty-eight, Nick was preparing to move to Colorado the following day. He was diagnosed as bipolar as a teen. He was brilliant and so kind toward his nephew Joe, who was born with Cerebral Palsy. Bless them as one day we shall be reunited.

Along with spontaneous adventures, I have been forced to take a look at my accumulated lifelong patterns of resistance, control, and fretting over what tomorrow may bring. Fortunately, I have had some excellent tools to assist me through these uncertain times. At a garage sale I bought *The Laws of Spirit* by Dan Millman. The story is about a man who meets a sage while on his mountain walk.

The woman teaches him about compassion, patience, balance, choices, faith, integrity, and surrender. Relevant for all of our lives, I believe. I also have been listening to the teachings of Abraham channeled through Esther Hicks. Abraham frequently uses the metaphor of paddling your boat downstream instead of bucking the current. Abraham also teaches that what we believe, we become, thus the law of attraction.

This book has been a labor of love which I tucked away in my mind for a very long time. I wrote it to share my life's experiences in health and mindfulness as well as guideposts for everyday living. The book shares many healthy ways to live through the foods we eat, our sense of purpose in life, and how we can continually improve each day as we age. I hope that the information has been valuable in your path to wholeness through body, mind, and spirit.

There are only two ways to live your life—one is as though nothing is a miracle; the other is as though everything is a miracle.

—Albert Einstein

A healthy lifestyle can be quite simply described, and you've no doubt heard much of it before. It may not be so easy to do: Love yourself. Keep fit. Move and stretch regularly in a way that feels right for you. Eat the right foods in moderation. Love yourself. Avoid that which is possibly harmful. Stay focused in the present and think positive, peaceful thoughts. Learn to acknowledge and express all your emotions and quickly release them. Love yourself. Laugh a lot. Cultivate and honor your intuition. Give yourself the gift of regular solitude, preferably in a natural environment. Be honest—especially with yourself. Love yourself. Reduce stress through a practice of regular meditation, intentional loving, allowing, and detachment. Reconnect with your Creator, your higher self, by consciously cultivating faith, hope, trust, and surrender. Learn to live with reverence and gratitude. But most of all, love yourself. Life always presents opportunities to reinvent ourselves. My grandchildren call me "Nonna"—Italian for grandmother. For now I have indeed become the Nonna who waits enthusiastically for the next voyage in my life. There are buckets of laughter with friends and family along with warm hugs from my many grandchildren.

For a long time it seemed to me that life was about to begin. Real life. But there was always some obstacle in the way, something to be gotten through first, some unfinished business, time still to be served, a debt to be paid. At last it dawned on me that these obstacles were my life. This perspective has helped me to see there is no way to happiness. Happiness is the way. So treasure every moment you have and remember that time waits for no one. Happiness is a journey, not a destination.

—Alfred D. Souza

Resources

Barrow, Becky. 2008. *Over-50s forced back to work to meet rising bills*. https://www.dailymail.co.uk/news/article-514299/Over-50s-forced-work-meet-rising-bills.html.

Emoto, Masaru. 2001. *The Hidden Messages in Water*. New York: Astria Books.

Erb and Erb. 2003. *The Slow Poisoning of America* (Paladins Press).

Goldberg, Elkhonon. 2006. *How Your Mind Can Grow Stronger As Your Brain Grows Older* (Penguin Publishing Group).

Hayley J. Koslik, Gavin Hamilton, Beatrice A. Golomb, Mitochondrial Dysfunction in Gulf War Illness Revealed by 31Phosphorus Magnetic Resonance Spectroscopy: A Case-Control Study. PLoS ONE, 2014; 9 (3): e92887 DOI: 10.1371/journal.pone.009288, University of California, San Diego Health Sciences

Lipton, Bruce. 2005. *The Biology of Belief.* US: Hay House, Inc.

Lloyd, Robin. 2006. *The Keys to Happiness, and Why We Don't Use Them*. https://www.livescience.com/7059-keys-happiness.html.

Orlando, James. 2023. The Greying of Canada's Population. https://economics.td.com/ca-demographics#:~:text=The%20Labour%20Force%20Survey%20estimates,older%20grow%20by%201%20million.

Plasker, Eric. 2007. *The 100 Year Lifestyle*. Adams Media Corp.

Tuttle, Dave, and Jack LaLanne. 2006. *"Godfather of Fitness" Still Going Strong at 91*. https://pals2u.tripod.com/id31.html.

University of Virginia Health System. 2015. "Missing Link Found Between Brain, Immune System." *Newsroom*. https://newsroom.uvahealth.com/2015/06/01/brain-immune-system-link/.

University of Virginia Health System. 2015. "Missing link found between brain, immune system; major disease implications." *Science News*. https://www.sciencedaily.com/releases/2015/06/150601122445.htm.

Vaughan, Christopher. 2016. *Researchers devise method for bone marrow transplants without using chemotherapy*. https://med.stanford.edu/news/all-news/2016/08/researchers-devise-safer-method-for-bone-marrow-transplants.html.

About the Author

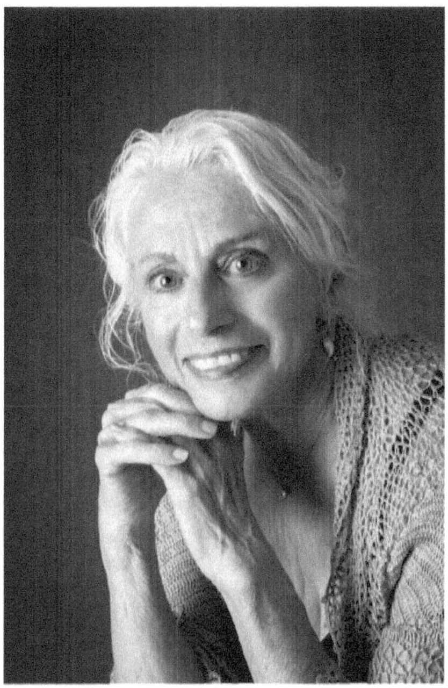

Cynthia Olsen {pen name} is the author of several books as well as founder of Kali Press in 1990. Ms. Olsen began writing books on health in 1989.

Her company is committed to writing on natural healing as well as healthy aging and spirituality.

In addition to her role as mother to her five children and her role as Nonna to her eight grandchildren and two great-grandchildren, Cynthia is a lifelong supporter of holistic living.

Cynthia studied and practiced yoga at an early age and continues her practice to this day. She has also practiced the Tibetan Five Rites and researched herbs, natural medicine, exercise, and is a strong believer in healing through the mind. She meditates, dances, swims, hikes, and brings joy and gratitude into her daily life.

Cynthia donated Essiac herbs to the Hopis on Second Mesa in Arizona. Her books have received recognition and awards. Now in her seventies, because of her appetite for continued learning and healthy lifestyle choices, she has amassed a wealth of information which she willingly shares through her writings and speaking engagements.

Learn how to Live Luminescently by visiting:

www.cynthiaolsen.com

For more books by Cynthia Olsen visit:

www.cynthiabelliniolsen.com

You can also reach Cynthia in her Facebook group or contact her directly with her author email.

www.facebook.com/cynthiaolsenauthor

author@cynthiaolsen.com

For more great books from Peak Press
Visit Books.GracePointPublishing.com

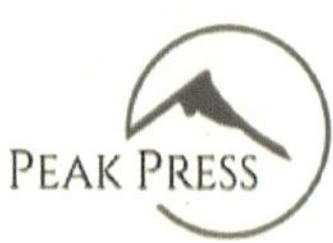

If you enjoyed reading *Embracing Your Age: Feeling Vibrant at Every Stage of Your Life* and purchased it through an online retailer, please return to the site and write a review to help others find the book.

www.ingramcontent.com/pod-product-compliance
Lightning Source LLC
LaVergne TN
LVHW091028080826
845145LV00002B/399

* 9 7 8 0 9 8 9 3 3 3 6 1 0 *